# CONTENTS

NEW DEVELOPMENTS IN MEDICAL RESEARCH

# STREPTOZOTOCIN

# USES, MECHANISM OF ACTION AND SIDE EFFECTS

# NEW DEVELOPMENTS IN MEDICAL RESEARCH

Additional books in this series can be found on Nova's website
under the Series tab.

Additional e-books in this series can be found on Nova's website
under the e-book tab.

NEW DEVELOPMENTS IN MEDICAL RESEARCH

# STREPTOZOTOCIN

## USES, MECHANISM OF ACTION AND SIDE EFFECTS

ELIZABETH L. GAUTHIER
EDITOR

New York

For permission to use material from this book please contact us:
Telephone 631-231-7269; Fax 631-231-8175
Web Site: http://www.novapublishers.com



**Library of Congress Cataloging-in-Publication Data**

ISBN: 978-1-63117-255-7

Library of Congress Control Number: 2014931438

*Published by Nova Science Publishers, Inc. † New York*

# PREFACE

Streptozotocin (STZ), an antibiotic and anticancer agent, is the most prominent diabetogenic chemical agent in diabetes research due to its cytotoxicity in pancreatic beta-cells. The selective toxicity of STZ to beta cells occurs because of its preferential accumulation in beta cells through uptake via GLUT2 glucose transporter. Insulin dependent diabetes mellitus can be induced by either single high dose or multiple low- dose STZ injections. At low dose, STZ induces pancreatic beta-cell apoptosis and at high dose it causes necrosis. Though STZ itself can cause carcinogenesis and renal, hepatic and muscle myoblast toxicity, these side effects can be minimized or completely avoided by using lower doses. This book discusses in further detail the different ways in which streptozotocin is used in the medical field.

Chapter 1 - Alzheimer's disease (AD) is the most common cause of dementia and leads to irreversible cognitive and memory impairment. By 2050 more than a 100 million people are expected to be affected by AD. Furthermore, AD cannot be prevented, it has no successful treatment and the ultimate neurotoxic mechanisms have not been completely elucidated. Pathological hallmarks of AD include: neurofibrillary tangles, which are intraneuronal deposits composed primarily of abnormally-phosphorylated tau protein; extracellular senile plaques, mainly composed of beta-amyloid peptide (Aβ), and neuronal and synaptic loss. On the other hand vascular dementia (VaD) is the second cause of dementia, and comprises a great variety of pathological features, including small vessel disease or white matter alterations, among others. Moreover the borderlines between AD and VaD are blurred and in many patients coexist simultaneously. In order to study the onset, evolution and therapeutic alternatives to treat AD, many transgenic mice engineered to overproduce Aβ or increase tau phosphorylation have been developed although only about 5-10% of the cases are familiar AD patients. On the other hand whereas age remains the main risk factor to suffer AD and VaD, multiple epidemiological studies reveal that diabetes mellitus is also a risk factor to suffer these diseases. In this sense streptozotocin (STZ) has been largely used for the last four decades as a pharmacological approach to induce type 1 diabetes (T1D) in rodents, and to study related metabolic alterations as well as the effect of different therapeutic agents. However in recent years central complications associated with diabetes are getting a great deal of attention, and central neuronal abnormalities, learning and memory impairment, central vascular dysfunction or blood brain barrier alterations have been observed after systemic administration of STZ. Moreover central administration of STZ, by icv injection, has been used as a model of sporadic AD to induce central alterations, such as tau phosphorylation, neurodegeneration, blood brain barrier dysfunction or cognitive impairment, as observed in AD and VaD patients. Taking into account these considerations in this study the authors will review recent literature where central alterations, resembling AD and VaD, have been described, both after systemic and central administration of STZ, and the authors will analyze the utility of STZ as a model of sporadic AD.

Chapter 2 - Streptozotocin (STZ), an antibiotic and anticancer agent, is the most prominent diabetogenic chemical agent in diabetes research due to its cytotoxicity to the pancreatic beta-cells. The selective toxicity of STZ to beta cells occurs because of its preferential accumulation in beta cells through uptake via GLUT2 glucose transporter. Insulin dependent diabetes mellitus can be induced by either single high dose or multiple low- dose STZ injections. At low dose, STZ induces pancreatic beta-cell apoptosis and at high dose it causes necrosis. The methylnitrosourea moiety derived from STZ has alkylating properties and is thought to modify macromolecules and break DNA strands which depletes the intracellular $NAD^+$ levels and inhibits beta cell function and insulin secretion. STZ also provokes oxidative stress that further contributes to beta cell toxicity. Though STZ itself can cause carcinogenesis and renal, hepatic and muscle myoblast toxicity, these side effects can be minimized or completely avoided by using lower doses. In addition, changes observed weeks after diabetes induction are less likely to result from direct effects of STZ as confirmed in spontaneous diabetic models. For example, multiple low-dose STZ induced diabetic rodent models display bone loss and show similar body parameters changes as spontaneous diabetic mouse models and diabetic patients. It is for this reason that STZ has been wildly used and serves as useful tools to examine mechanisms of type 1 diabetes and its complications.

Chapter 3 - Diabetes mellitus is a common and growing metabolic disorder that is associated with chronic complications, particularly affecting kidney, vessels and neural tissues. Cell targets in the central nervous system include neurons and astrocytes. Brain commitment has been confirmed by cognitive impairment in the diabetic population and experimental models of diabetes.

In addition, the authors know that the risk for Alzheimer′s disease is increased in diabetic individuals. Glucosamine-nitrosourea streptozotocin (STZ) administration has been widely used to induce experimental diabetes, due to its toxicity to β-cells of the islets of Langerhans.

This compound does not cross the blood brain barrier, but the brain damage associated with ensuing diabetes can, therefore, be studied. Conversely, intracerebroventricular injection of STZ has been used as a model of dementia, where many characteristics of Alzheimer′s disease are observed to include β-amyloid deposits. In this chapter, the authors will discuss the link between the cognitive impairment in diabetes mellitus and Alzheimer′s disease, using the experimental evidence obtained using STZ administration and focusing on the alterations in astrocytes, the most abundant glial cells that are intimately connected (both structurally and metabolically) to neurons.

Chapter 4 - Type 1 and type 2 diabetes mellitus (DM) are characterized by hyperglycemia, due to lost or damaged insulin-producing β-cells within the pancreatic islets of Langerhans. Rodent models of DM result in hyperglycemia, arising from different forms of islet deterioration. Streptozotocin (STZ) is currently used to induce experimental DM in rodents because it selectively targets pancreatic β-cells. STZ enters β-cells via a glucose transporter (GLUT2), causing DNA alkylation, which in turn activates poly ADP-ribosylation, leading to ATP depletion and resulting in the formation of superoxide anions. Concomitantly, STZ triggers nitric oxide formation, which results in DNA damage. Both of these actions cause β-cell necrosis, leading to DM. These features provide a methodological advantage for STZ, resulting in the development of human-like DM. However, there is no consensus across the literature regarding the optimal STZ dose or administration route for developing rodent models of DM. In addition, the nutritional status of the animals employed has also been shown to influence outcomes. This review aims to compare the different methodologies, considering their advantages and disadvantages.

Chapter 5 - *M*atrix *m*etallo*p*roteases (MMPs) are a family of metal ion-dependent extracellular matrix (ECM) degrading enzymes that play crucial roles in tissue remodeling and repair, and may be involved in the development and progression of diabetic complications.

The most frequent complications in diabetes mellitus are consequences of macro- and microangiopathies, which affect many organs and tissues. Diabetic macroangiopathy manifests as an atherosclerosis-like condition, characterized by formation of plaques that follows an accelerated course, and diabetic microangiopathy is characterized by progressive arteriolosclerosis and interstitial fibrosis, with ECM accumulation and changes in its quality, as well as basement membrane thickening. These are structural hallmarks in all organs affected by diabetic complications, and may occur in response to insults such as hyperglycemia and hypertension.

A few examples illustrate the relevance of MMPs in diabetic complications: regarding cardiovascular system, it was shown that inhibition of MMP-2 and MMP-9 ameliorates cardiovascular dysfunction, becoming a possible therapeutic target; in diabetic brain, increased MMP activities (especially MMP-9) were reported, possibly contributing to blood-brain barrier degradation and cognitive impairment; increased MMP-9 occurs in diabetic skin, especially around wounds, and its expression was inhibited by siRNA, maybe providing a new therapeutic approach for diabetic skin wounds; MMP-2 and MMP-9 activities were shown to be increased in sera and placentas of diabetic rats, and both decreased when the animals were treated with dietary olive and safflower oils; in diabetic nephropathy, the accumulation of ECM leads to glomerulosclerosis, interstitial fibrosis, tubular atrophy, and finally renal failure, and MMPs may be involved; recent evidences suggest that diabetes is a risk factor for the development of progressive liver disease, including non-alcoholic steatohepatitis, cirrhosis, and primary liver cancer. *In vitro* studies have shown that high glucose concentration can alter the expression of some MMPs (and also their endogenous inhibitors, TIMPs), and this effect might be mediated by connective tissue growth factor.

Hence, the aim of the present paper is to set the stage for a better understanding of the role of MMPs in streptozotocin-induced diabetes mellitus, focusing the main targets of diabetic complications: heart, brain, skin, uterus, kidney, and liver. In addition to discussing the literature, unpublished results on kidney and liver are also given.

Chapter 6 - Streptozotocin (Streptozocin, STZ, CAS No. 18883-66-4) is a monofunctional nitrosourea derivative isolated from *Streptomyces achromogenes* with broad spectrum antibiotic activity and antineoplastic properties. This compound is often used to induce diabetes *mellitus* in experimental animals through its toxic effects on pancreatic β-cells. STZ is a potent alkylating agent known to directly methylate DNA, thus inducing DNA damage by alkylation of specific sites on DNA bases. DNA lesions produced by STZ includes double and single-strand breaks, covalent adducts and alkali-labile sites. Moreover, STZ induces unscheduled DNA synthesis and DNA synthesis inhibition. Severe DNA damage by STZ results in cell death by apoptosis or necrosis. The DNA strand breaks resulting from the alkylating action of STZ can lead to chromosomal rearrangements. Accordingly, STZ tests positive in the chromosomal aberrations, micronuclei and sister chromatid exchanges assays. In addition, this antibiotic was found to be mutagenic in bacterial assays and eukaryotic cells and is also carcinogenic: a single administration of STZ induces tumors in rat kidney, liver, and pancreas. Since STZ is used as an antineoplastic agent for the treatment of pancreatic neuroendocrine carcinomas, the study of its genotoxicity is of great importance to understand the genomic instability associated with chemotherapy regimens involving administration of this antibiotic. Therefore, the purpose of this chapter is to summarize the current knowledge regarding the genotoxic effects of STZ.

Chapter 7 - Streptozotocin (STZ: 2-deoxy-2-(3-(methyl-3-nitrosoureido)-D-glucopyranose) is synthesized by *Streptomycetes achromogenes* and is used to induce both insulin-dependent and non-insulin-dependent diabetes mellitus (IDDM and NIDDM, respectively).

The single intravenous dose most frequently used in adult rats to induce IDDM is between 40 and 60 mg/kg b.w., but higher doses are also used. STZ is also efficacious after intraperitoneal administration of a similar or higher dose.

Streptozotocin action on B cells is accompanied by characteristic alterations in the blood levels of insulin and glucose. Two hours after injection, hyperglycemia is observed together with a concomitant drop in blood insulin. About six hours later, hypoglycemia occurs with high levels of blood insulin. Finally, hyperglycemia develops and blood insulin levels decrease. These changes in the blood levels of glucose and insulin reflect abnormalities of B cell function. STZ impairs glucose oxidation and decreases insulin biosynthesis and secretion.

The liver plays an important role in the metabolism and excretion of STZ. At first, the authors analyzed the direct effect of STZ on the hepatobiliary function. The effect of streptozotocin on hepatobiliary function was studied in rats on the 1$^{st}$, 7$^{th}$ and 15$^{th}$ days after treatment. Serum glucose significantly increased on the 1st day, and remained high onwards. Bile flow and the bile acids output were significantly decreased on the 1$^{st}$ day of treatment. Also, the biliary excretion of sulfobromophthalein (BSP, a substance used for evaluating the function of the liver) was significantly decreased on the first day of treatment. All parameters tested, except for serum glucose, tended to normalize at 7$^{th}$ day after treatment. The results suggested a transient toxic effect of STZ on the hepatocyte. It is known that bile flow (BF) is determined by two fractions: the bile acid dependent flow (BADF) and the bile acid independent flow (BAIF). The authors analyzed both fractions and demonstrated that STZ itself, and not its diabetogenic effect, produced a diminution in BF at the expense of both BAIF and BADF.

In a second stage, the authors used STZ to induce insulin-dependent diabetes in rats. It is known that the liver is a central regulator of carbohydrate homeostasis and it releases glucose according to metabolic demand. Besides, in the last years, liver injury has been recognized as a major complication of diabetes mellitus (DM).

The authors analyzed the contribution of oxidative stress and Tumor Necrosis Factor alpha (TNF-$\alpha$) intracellular pathway in the development of apoptosis in the liver of streptozotocin- induced diabetic animals. In this review, the authors describe the role of upstream mediators of the interaction between TNF$\alpha$ and its receptor, TNFR1, by assessing the ability of the *in vivo* treatment with etanercept (TNF-$\alpha$ blocking antibody) to protect against TNF-$\alpha$-induced apoptosis. Also, the authors studied the role of iNOS-induction in the

TNF-α pathways of liver apoptosis in IDDM, by treatment of diabetic rats with aminoguanidine (selective iNOS inhibitor), which blocked the induction of apoptosis. Interestingly, iNOS inhibition significantly reduced TNF-α levels, thus evidencing an interaction between TNF-α and iNOS activity. On the other hand, the authors found that the administration of antioxidants/hydroxyl radical scavengers (Tempol and Desferal) prevented oxidative stress by reducing the effects of hydroxyl radical production and both LPO levels and apoptosis. Taken together, the author's studies support the notion that, at least in part, the hydroxyl radical acts as a reactive intermediate, which leads to liver apoptosis in a model of STZ-mediated hyperglycemia.

The present review bears two major insights:

First, it provides evidence for a transient toxic effect of STZ on the hepatobiliary function. This toxic effect becomes relevant for the study, at short time, of hepatic metabolism in the experimental diabetes induced by STZ.

Second, it provides further knowledge about the mechanisms which may contribute to the disease process in the liver during the course of an inflammatory process as is IDDM. Regulation of hepatic oxidative stress and TNF-α levels in the diabetic state could be of therapeutic relevance for the improvement or delay of the hepatic complications linked to chronic hyperglycemia.

In: Streptozotocin: Uses, Mechanism of Action and Side Effects ISBN: 978-1-63117-255-7
Editor: Elizabeth L. Gauthier 

*Chapter 1*

# STREPTOZOTOCIN AS A TOOL TO INDUCE CENTRAL PATHOLOGY AND COGNITIVE IMPAIRMENT IN RODENTS

*Monica Garcia-Alloza*[*]
Division of Physiology. School of Medicine
University of Cadiz, Cádiz, Spain

## ABSTRACT

Alzheimer's disease (AD) is the most common cause of dementia and leads to irreversible cognitive and memory impairment. By 2050 more than a 100 million people are expected to be affected by AD. Furthermore, AD cannot be prevented, it has no successful treatment and the ultimate neurotoxic mechanisms have not been completely elucidated. Pathological hallmarks of AD include: neurofibrillary tangles, which are intraneuronal deposits composed primarily of abnormally-phosphorylated tau protein; extracellular senile plaques, mainly composed of beta-amyloid peptide (Aβ), and neuronal and synaptic loss. On the other hand vascular dementia (VaD) is the second cause of dementia, and comprises a great variety of pathological features, including small vessel disease or white matter alterations, among others. Moreover the borderlines between AD and VaD are blurred and in many patients coexist simultaneously. In order to study the onset, evolution and therapeutic alternatives to treat AD, many transgenic mice engineered to overproduce Aβ or increase tau phosphorylation have been developed although only about 5-10% of the cases are familiar AD patients. On the other hand whereas age remains the main risk factor to suffer AD and VaD, multiple epidemiological studies reveal that diabetes mellitus is also a risk factor to suffer these diseases. In this sense streptozotocin (STZ) has been largely used for the last four decades as a pharmacological approach to induce type 1 diabetes (T1D) in rodents, and to study related metabolic alterations as well as the effect of different therapeutic agents. However in recent years central complications associated with diabetes are getting a great deal of attention, and central neuronal abnormalities, learning and memory impairment, central vascular dysfunction or blood brain barrier alterations have been observed after

[*] Corresponding author: Monica Garcia-Alloza, PhD. Division of Physiology, School of Medicine. University of Cadiz. Plaza Fragela 9, 4 piso, 410. Cadiz (11003). Tel: +34 956015252. Email: monica.garcia@uca.es.

systemic administration of STZ. Moreover central administration of STZ, by icv injection, has been used as a model of sporadic AD to induce central alterations, such as tau phosphorylation, neurodegeneration, blood brain barrier dysfunction or cognitive impairment, as observed in AD and VaD patients. Taking into account these considerations in this study we will review recent literature where central alterations, resembling AD and VaD, have been described, both after systemic and central administration of STZ, and we will analyze the utility of STZ as a model of sporadic AD.

# 1. INTRODUCTION

## 1.1. Alzheimer's Disease

Alzheimer's disease (AD) is the most common cause of dementia, accounting for ~50-70% of all dementia cases, and leads to irreversible cognitive and memory impairment. In 2006 about 26.6 million people suffered from AD all over the world, with an associated cost of ~220 million euros (Wimo et al., 2006), and in 2050 more than a 100 million people are expected to be affected by AD (Brookmeyer et al., 2007). Neuropathological features include: 1) neurofibrillary tangles, 2) senile plaques and 3) synaptic loss (Hyman & Trojanowski 1997). Neurofibrilary tangles are intraneuronal deposits composed primarily by abnormally phosphorylated tau protein. Tau is phosphorylated at different sites as disease progresses and phosphorylation state of tau results from a coordinated balance between kinase-mediated phosphorylations of tau and dephosphorylation by protein phosphatases (Clodfelder-Miller et al., 2006), that leads to neurofibrillary tangle formation and deposition. Tau deposition increases in parallel with the duration and severity of the illness (Hyman & Gomez-Isla 1996), however previous studies also indicate that neurofibrillary tangles are the latest pathological feature in the development of the illness (Woodhouse et al., 2005, Gong et al., 2010). Senile plaques, mainly composed by peptide beta-amyloid (Aβ), are a pathological feature extremely frequent in AD brains although Aβ can also deposit as cerebral amyloid angiopathy (CAA) surrounding brain vessels. Aβ is a 39-43 aminoacid peptide derived of the progressive cleavage of the Aβ precursor protein (APP) by β and γ secretases. Pathology and, dynamic formation and remodelation of senile plaques, as well as the specific implication of Aβ are not fully understood, although Aβ in different aggregation states, as well as compact senile plaques, are neurotoxic both in AD and experimental animal models (Urbanc et al., 2002), and they have been suggested to induce synaptic loss and dystrophic neurites (Brendza et al., 2005, Larson et al., 1999, Lombardo et al., 2003). Senile plaques have also been associated with abnormal neuritic curvature (Craft 2009, Knowles et al., 1999, Meyer-Luehmann et al., 2008, Spires et al., 2005) and may alter cortical synaptic integration (Stern et al., 2004). Neuronal loss is the pathological feature that best correlates with duration and severity of the illness. In this sense neuronal loss of >50% is observed in the associative cortex in AD patients (for review see (Serrano-Pozo et al., 2011, Gomez-Isla et al., 1997).

Although the ultimate neurotoxic mechanisms have not been completely elucidated recent evidence supports a biphasic evolution of AD, including an amyloid dependent and amyloid-independent stages of AD. Following this idea in an initial phase disruption of the neuropil, loss of dendritic spines, remodelling of neurites, and inflammatory responses would derive from soluble oligomeric and fibrilar Aβ accumulation, the second phase would consist of the further development of tangles, synaptic and neuronal loss (Hyman 2011). At present AD has no successful treatment and current pharmacological approaches are limited to anticholinesterase drugs, such as donezepil, and glutamatergic antagonists like memantin. On the other hand active Aβ imunization has been widely explored, and senile plaques and Aβ remain a major therapeutic target, however the incidence of meningoencephalitis in AD immunized patients (6%) has significantly limited this approach (Orgogozo et al., 2003). At this point we cannot obviate that senile plaques and Aβ levels only characterize parts of a complex combination of pathological features, and the presence of soluble microscopic oligomeric forms of Aβ, could underlined cognitive alterations (He et al., 2013), since they likely contribute to the progressive neural system failure that occurs over decades (Serrano-Pozo et al., 2011).

Mutations of APP, or the proteolytic enzymes that generate Aβ, presenilins 1 and 2, are responsible for most of the familiar AD cases. However the vast majority of AD cases (~95%) are sporadic (Harman 2006) and the ultimate causes have not been elucidated. Following this idea heterogeneous associated aspects and pathological features have been observed among patients (Bhat 2010) and, although age remains the main risk factor to suffer dementia, recent studies have focused on metabolic alterations such as hypertension (de Leeuw et al., 2002, Reitz et al., 2007), hypercholesterolemia (Pappolla 2008, Pappolla et al., 2003), hyperhomocysteinemia (Seshadri et al., 2002) or arteriosclerosis-related factors (Honig et al., 2005). Interestingly, hyperinsulinemia and diabetes display a strong association with dementia (Luchsinger et al., 2004, Schrijvers et al., 2010) and the risk factor to suffer AD seem to largely increase in diabetic patients (Craft 2009).

## 1.2. Vascular Dementia

Vascular dementia (VaD) has been traditionally considered the second most common cause of progressive and irreversible dementia; although Lewy body dementia is also considered the second leading cause of dementia by some experts (Gorelick & Nyenhuis 2013). VaD is an heterogeneous pathology that can range from multiple microinfacts to small vessel ischemic disease or to microvascular injury (Craft 2009, O'Brien 2006), all of which might be triggered and have been associated with Aβ deposition as CAA in cerebral blood vessels (Greenberg et al., 2008). Classification of VaD is based on clinical differences and pathological changes, however in practice it is difficult to classify a patient into a specific subtype of VaD, since they usually present mixtures or pathology that contribute to cognitive impairment (Chen et al., 2013a, Moorhouse & Rockwood 2008). The borderlines between AD and VaD are thus blurred and in many patients markers of vascular injury coexist with traditional AD hallmarks. Furthermore strokes and AD often occur concomitantly and pose risks for one another (Gorelick & Nyenhuis 2013). Folowing this idea, considerable evidence indicates that stroke increases the risk of dementia (Ivan et al., 2004). In some cases AD features might be promoted by a specific form of vascular injury; for example blood brain barrier dysfunction may affect Aβ transport between brain and periphery, and thereby contribute to parenchymal and neurovascular Aβ deposition (Craft 2009). On the other hand AD pathology may cause vascular injury, as when Aβ-induced inflammation damages the endothelium. The pathological consequences of vascular damage include alteration of functional markers, such as increased reactive oxygen species (ROS) or increased matrix-metalloproteinases (MMPs) activity (Garcia-Alloza et al., 2009). All these processes have been related in a different extent to neuronal death (Brown et al., 2009, Zhang & Murphy 2007). Although the ultimate cause of VaD is not clear, many studies have pointed out the significant effect of metabolic disorders on VaD, and type 2 diabetes (T2D) might play a significant role at this level (for review see (Gorelick 2004, Roman 2005, Craft 2009)).

### 1.3. Diabetes Mellitus

Diabetes mellitus is one of the most prevalent diseases in western countries. The total number of people with diabetes is projected to rise from 171 million in 2000 to 366 million in 2030 (Wild et al., 2004). Type 1 diabetes (T1D) is a autoimmune disease characterized by pancreatic β-cells apoptosis, lack of insulin and hyperglicemia (Lee 2013) however about 90% of all the cases are type 2 diabetes (T2D) (Gotz et al., 2009). Since T2D prevalence increases with age, the progressive aging of population seems to indicate that the "diabetes epidemic" will continue (Wild et al., 2004). T2D is characterized by an initial stage of insulin resistance and hyperglycaemia. In order to compensate this deficit, β-pancreatic cells respond by increasing insulin production. Insulin secretion occurs in tandem with amylin, also implicated in the control of glucose levels. When β-pancreatic cells are exhausted and can no longer overproduce insulin, T2D evolves. T2D is associated with other peripheral alterations such as hypertension, cardiovascular disease, dyslipidemia or hypercholesterolemia, that have been addressed in detail both in basic science studies (Jelinek et al., 2011, Russell & Proctor 2006) and in epidemiological and clinical studies (35; 37). In recent years more and more studies have focused on the relationship between diabetes and central nervous systems alterations, with special interest in neurodegeneration and dementia, although the mechanisms implicated have not been elucidated.

## 2. Link Between Diabetes and Alzheimer´s Disease and Vascular Dementia

Association between T2D and dementia has been studied in the last decades and in the Rotterdam study Ott et al., (Ott et al., 1996) observed that T2D patients had a relative risks of 1.4 to suffer AD, duplicating this value in case of VaD. Other epidemiological studies have supported these data (Luchsinger et al., 2004, Plastino et al., 2010). It also seems that a combination of vascular risk factors, such as heart disease, hyperlipidemia, hypercholesterolemia, smoking, or more relevantly T2D, increase the risk to suffer AD (Luchsinger et al., 2005). Moreover, insulin levels and insulin resistance seem to be the parameters that best correlate with a higher risk to develop AD (Schrijvers et al., 2010). On the other hand mouse models of T1D also display similar patterns of peripheral neuropathy, with decreased motor nerve conduction velocity, to those observed in AD models (Jolivalt et al., 2012). Some relevant links between diabetes and AD have contributed to the association of both pathologies and the description of a complex syndrome defined as type 3 diabetes (T3D) (de la Monte & Wands 2008, Steen et al., 2005). Among others: 1) Early studies by Frolich et al., (Frolich et al., 1998) showed that brain insulin receptor densities were altered in sporadic AD patients. Further studies have confirmed these findings, and extensive abnormalities in insulin and insulin-like growth factor (IGF) type 1 (IGF-1) and 2 (IGF-2) signaling mechanisms have been documented (Steen et al., 2005). 2) Central nervous system insulin receptors, located in astrocytes and neuronal synapses, are highly expressed in the basal forebrain, origin of the cortical and hippocampal cholinergic innervation. Cholinergic system seems to be of special vulnerability in AD, and cholinergic loss of the basal forebrain seems to be a good predictor of the clinical dementia in AD (Roberson & Harrell 1997, Schliebs & Arendt 2006, Walsh & Selkoe 2004). On the other hand insulin receptors are also expressed in relevant regions for learning and memory, such as cortex and hippocampus. This is consistent with evidence showing that insulin influences memory (Craft 2009), likely due to modulation of synaptic structure and function, long-term potentiation and central nervous system levels of neurotransmitters such as acetylcholine, of special relevance in AD (Roberson & Harrell 1997, Schliebs & Arendt 2006). 3) T2D progression correlates with pancreatic amylin deposition, in a similar way to Aβ deposition in AD brains. Moreover insulin, amylin and Aβ are degraded by neprelysin (NEP) and insulin degrading enzyme (IDE), and both NEP and IDE substrates can compete with each other. It has been postulated that an imbalance of substrates can affect the degradation rate of other substrates and possibly influence the pathogenesis of AD and T2D (Gotz et al., 2009). Following this idea it has been shown that insulin increases extracellular Aβ, both by increasing its secretion and by inhibiting its degradation by IDE (Qiu et al., 1998, Vekrellis et al., 2000). 4) Postmortem studies in human AD brains have shown reduced expression of the insulin protein and its mRNA levels, accompanied by reductions of IGF genes as well as their corresponding receptors (Lester-Coll et al., 2006, Steen et al., 2005). 5) Aβ oligomers may interfere insulin signaling in hippocampal neurons (Zhao et al., 2008). On the other hand insulin may regulate Aβ levels by modulation of β and γ secretases (Eckman & Eckman 2005, Farris et al., 2003). Accordingly, reduced brain insulin signaling increases Aβ levels in a mouse model of T1D (Jolivalt et al., 2008). 6) Also insulin seems to participate in cerebrovascular regulation by multiple mechanisms, including endothelium-dependent mechanisms, nitric oxide or cyclooxygenase activity, among others, linking metabolic disorders with VaD associated pathology (Correia et al., 2011). 7) Extensive evidence supports Aβ toxicity in different states of aggregation (Frydman-Marom et al., 2011, Meyer-Luehmann et al., 2008, Spires et al., 2005, Urbanc et al., 2002, Yao et al., 2011) and it seems that amylin, similarly to Aβ, can induce apoptotic cell death (Konarkowska et al., 2006, Matveyenko & Butler 2006). It is likely that amylin and Aβ aggregates alter cellular function by similar mechanisms, such as inducing ROS (Craft 2009). Following this idea hyperglycemia enhances the formation of advanced glycation end products, which by interacting with their receptor elicits the formation of ROS, that are also believed to be an early event in AD pathology (Guglielmotto et al., 2012). 8) Insulin has also been linked to tau phosphorylation, as a major pathological feature observed in AD, since insulin has been shown to activate kinases involved in tau phosphorylation such as GSK-3 (Yang et al., 2013b). Also, in a T1D animal model reduced brain insulin signaling results in increased tau hyperphosphorilation (Jolivalt et al., 2008). Altogether it seems clear that insulin plays a crucial role in maintaining brain normal activity, and alterations of insulin dependent functions could be associated with central pathological conditions, observed in sporadic AD and VaD (Correia et al., 2011, Craft 2009).

Overally, these data have lead to the description of a complex syndrome: type 3 diabetes mellitus (T3D) as a consequence of the relationship between T2D-AD-VaD (figure 1). Albeit all the circumstantial links mentioned above, experimental data supporting a direct relationship between T2D, EA and VaD are limited, mostly because 1) studying the mechanistic relationship of insulin resistance to AD and VaD is hampered by the complexity of its measurement, 2) animal models are limited, and 3) diabetes is a complex disorder and so it is likely that multiple different, synergistic processes may interact to promote cognitive impairment (Craft, 2009; Strachan et al., 2008). Therefore the vast majority of studies are epidemiological, in which T2D is identified as a risk factor to suffer AD or VaD (Luchsinger et al., 2005, Luchsinger et al., 2004, Matsuzaki et al., 2010, Schrijvers et al., 2010). It should also be pointed out that studies with T2D patients and clinical diagnosis of AD or VaD have faced some challenges (for review see Craft, 2009): patients with diabetes are often presumed to have dementia of vascular origin and the effects of treatments for T2D may affect AD markers and vascular integrity (Craft 2009). Therefore in order to accurately delineate the pathogenesis of cognitive impairment in people with T2D, large-scale, prospective epidemiological studies are still required (Strachan et al., 2008).

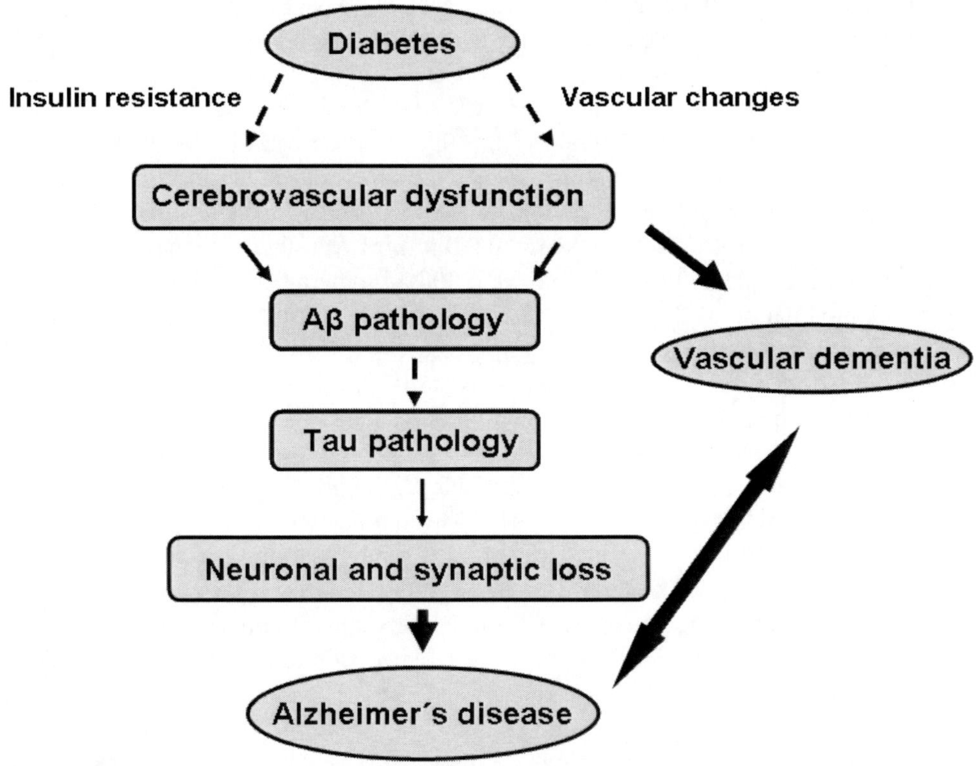


Figure 1. Schematic review or the relationship between diabetes, Alzheimer's disease and vascular dementia. Adapted from Bhat, 2010. © 2010 The Author. Journal of Neurochemistry © 2010 International Society for Neurochemistry.

## 3. Transgenic and Knock-Out Animal Models of Type 2 Diabetes, Alzheimer´S Disease and Vascular Dementia

To our knowledge, there are only a handful of studies where an effort has been made to set T2D and AD together. Takeda et al., (Takeda et al., 2010) have developed a mixed T2D and AD model, crossing a model of T2D: ob/ob mice (leptin-defficient mice) or NSY mice, and a model of AD: APP23 mice, that presents Aβ deposition with aging. This study supports the cross-talk between T2D and AD. T2D worsened cognitive performance as well as cerebrovascular inflamation and CAA in the generated mice, whereas parenchymal Aβ burden was not altered. On the other hand Takeda et al., (2011) also showed that AD may interfere with natural evolution of T2D, since cross-bred mice showed an accelerated diabetic phenotype compared with ob/ob mice, suggesting that cerebrovascular changes and alteration in brain insulin signaling might play a pivotal role in the relationship between T2D and AD. Whereas an extremely novedous and promising animal model, mice were used at relatively young ages and little is stated about long-term effects, while both T2D and AD are chronic diseases closely influenced by age. In fact APP23 mice need long life span to develop the illness. A recent study (Hiltunen et al., 2012) has also observed learning impairment in pancreatic IGF-2 overexpressing mice crossed with APPswe/PS1dE9 mice. APP/PS1 mice (Jankowsky et al., 2004) are a relevant and widely used model of AD, that shows robust Aβ deposition by 6 months of age (Garcia-Alloza et al., 2006b). However IGF-2 overexpressing mice are a limited model of T2D, since they display mild hyperglycemia, and only about 30% of the mice develop overt diabetes when fed a high fat diet (Devedjian et al., 2000). These aspects may account for the fact that significant characteristics of AD, such as Aβ burden, are not affected in IGF-2XAPP/PS1 mice (Hiltunen et al., 2012). Also a recent approach includes crossing db/db mice (leptin receptor KO mice) as a model of T2D with APPswe/PS1dE9 mice (Jimenez-Palomares et al., 2012). Although to our knowledge these mice have not have been characterized at central level, it seems that the presence of the APP/PS1 transgenes is enough to worsen metabolic parameters in heterozygous db/db mice, that otherwise would not present metabolic dysfunction.

Whereas extremely useful all these models are based on transgenic and knock-out mice and only a small number of AD cases (Serrano-Pozo et al., 2011) and diabetes, as well as associated metabolic alterations (Saxena et al., 2007, Weedon & Frayling 2007), are of familiar origin. Therefore exploring other animal models s might be of great value in the study of the relationship between diabetes, AD and VaD.

## 4. Pharmacological Model: Streptozotocin

Taking into account previous considerations, including the necessity to have animal models that reproduce sporadic AD, as well as the close relationship between T2D and AD-VaD, the use streptozotozin (STZ) (2-deoxy-2-(3-(methyl-3-nitrosoureido))-D-glucopyranose) might provide a different approach to address these aspects. STZ is a β-pancreatic cells toxin isolated from the bacterium Streptomycetes achromogens (Nugent et al., 2008). STZ has been classic pharmacological tool to induce in rodents both T1D and T2D, depending on the administration protocols used (Patel & Bhadada 2013, Ding et al., 2013, Clodfelder-Miller et al., 2006). In this sense peripheral administration at high doses completely destroys β-pancreatic cells, causing T1D, lower doses of STZ cause insulin resistance by damaging insulin receptors, resembling T2D (Salkovic-Petrisic et al., 2013a). It also seems that as a T2D models, a more complete version of the disease is observed when STZ is administered in combination with long-term high fat diet (Srinivasan et al., 2005, Zhang et al., 2008). It has been suggested that this might be more representative of westernized diet-associated diabetes, while an alternative to genetic models (Nugent et al., 2008). STZ has been widely used as a tool to induce diabetes, and central alterations associated to the model have also been observed, both after peripheral and central administration of the drug, resembling alterations observed in dementia processes, including AD and VaD. However it has been in the last two decades that central STZ has been considered as a suitable model for T3D, after icv injection (de la Monte & Wands 2008, Salkovic-Petrisic et al., 2013a).

### 4.1. Alzheimer´S Disease and Vascular Dementia-Like Complications Associated to Peripheral Administration of STZ

STZ has been a classical model to induce diabetes, therefore initial observations regarding central pathology respond to the peripheral administration of the drug used to induce T1 or T2D. STZ itself cannot pass through the blood-brain barrier due to the absence of the STZ transporter GLUT2 at this level. Therefore, the systemic-injection consequences relay on the effect of systemic hypoinsulinemia on the brain (Park 2011). Whereas outcomes at central level have been quite reproducible, many different administration protocols have been used in previous studies, ranging from various medium doses (50 mg/Kg) (Ramos-Rodriguez et al., 2013) to a single very high dose of STZ (70 mg/kg) (Revsin et al., 2009). As previously stated insulin resistant conditions do not only affect peripheral tissues, but also brain function can be significantly affected. In this sense original studies on brains from peripherally STZ injected mice already showed some pathological features, including focal accumulation of collagen fibrils in the basement membranes of arteriole and capillary walls (Mukai et al., 1980), similar to those observed in some variants of VaD in humans (Burke et al., 2013, Craggs et al., 2013). Following this idea, peripherally administered STZ also impairs endothelium function, and it has also been considered a model of VaD (Sharma & Singh 2011, Sharma & Singh 2010). More recently it has been observed that vascular alterations in C57Bl6 mice treated with STZ lead to spontaneous small vessel hemorrhages (Ramos-Rodriguez et al., 2013) as observed in figure 2, showing a severe case of VaD-like vascular dysfunction. On the other hand oxidative stress related macro and microgangiopathy may induce neuronal damage caused by chronic intracellular hyperglycaemia, leading to increased production of ROS in the brain, and reducing antioxidant capacity in STZ treated rats (Tahirovic et al., 2007) as observed in AD animal models and Alzheimer's patients (Dumont & Beal 2011, Garcia-Alloza et al., 2010, Garcia-Alloza et al., 2006a). Also, random degeneration of neuronic cells has been observed in STZ treated rats (Mukai et al., 1980) and a significant cortical atrophy has been observed in STZ treated mice (Ramos-Rodriguez et al., 2013), supporting similar findings to those detected in AD patients. In humans estimates of tissue damage, or loss in characteristically vulnerable brain regions, such as the hippocampus and entorhinal cortex are predictive of progression of middle cognitive impairment to AD (Frisoni et al., 2010).

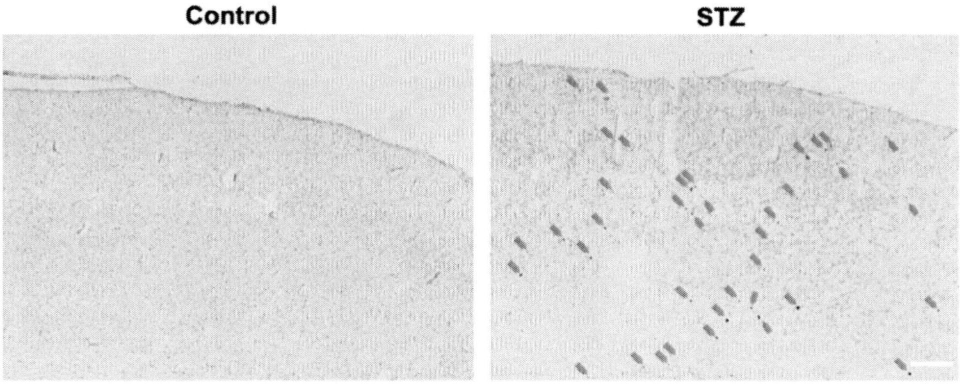


Figure 2. Illustrative example of the presence of hemorrhages in the cortex of C57Bl6 mice 8 weeks after ip STZ injection (50 mg/Kg, 5 consecutive days) stained with Prussian blue, and counterstained with neutral red. Green arrows point at hemorrhages and a great amount of spontaneous bleeding can be observed in STZ treated mice. Scale bar=250 μm.

Other studies have also reported that insulin deficiency, after STZ administration to amyloid models of AD may worsen AD-like pathological features. In this sense, STZ may accelerate amyloid pathology in APP mice, by increasing total Aβ levels and senile plaques deposition (Jolivalt et al., 2010). Further assessment in other AD mice have shown similar results, and increased senile plaques deposition has been observed in APP/PS1 mice as well as enhanced APP processing, including increased levels of APP695 protein, BACE1 and APP cleavage fragments (sAPPα, sAPPβ and CTFs) (Wang et al., 2010). A similar profile has been observed in 5xFAD mice, in which increased APP processing, due to higher BACE1 levels, has been observed accompanied by increased Aβ40 and Aβ42 levels (Devi et al., 2012). Also, in a mouse model presenting both Aβ and tau pathology (3xTg-AD mice) an increase in brain APP and Aβ levels was observed after peripheral STZ challenge (Li et al., 2010), supporting the capacity of STZ to interfere with APP processing.

When tau pathology has been assessed in AD mice after STZ treatment, slight differences have been observed among animal models. Whereas no effect was detected in 3xTg-AD mice (Li et al., 2010), a significant increase in tau phosphorylation at the threonine 231 site (part of the microtubule-binding domain), and at Ser199/202 (a marker for neurofibrilary tangles), has been observed, probably mediated by reduced GSK3β phosphorylation at the recognized inactivating site (ser 9) (Jolivalt et al., 2010). Tau hyperphosphorylation increases as disease progresses, in particular at pathologic sites, such as pS422, concomitant with neurofibrillary tangle formation. Increased tau phosphorylation at this residue has been observed in pR5 mice, that express the longest human tau isoform carrying the pathogenic P301L mutation (Ke et al., 2009). In this animal model a significant increase in pS422 phosphorylation was detected in the amygdala, indicating that more NFTs may have been induced by the STZ treatment than are normally found at this age. Further assessment of neurofibrillary tangles by Gallyas silver impregnation revealed advanced deposition of fibrillar tau in STZ-treated pR5 mice (Ke et al., 2009). Following this idea rats on high fat diet, high protein and high glucose diet, in combination with intraperitoneal injection of STZ presented an increase in tau hyperphosphorylation, decreased AKT activation, and GSK-3β over-activation (Yang et al., 2013a).

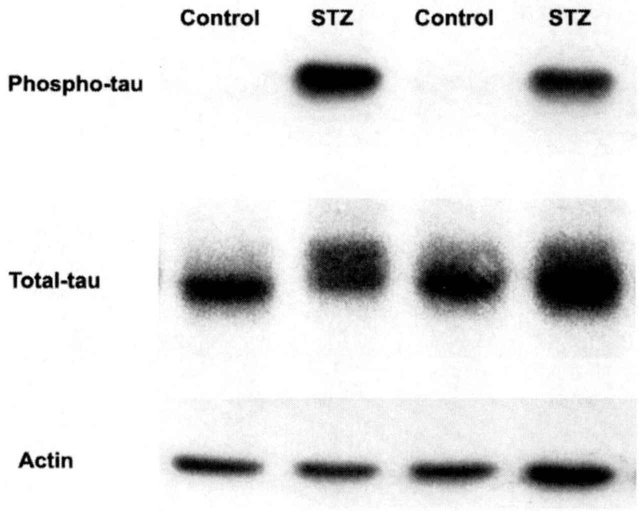


Figure 3. Example of cortical tau hyperphosphorylation by western blot in C57Bl6 mice, 8 weeks after ip STZ injection (50 mg/Kg, 5 consecutive days), using 4T8 antibody. Whereas total tau and actin levels remained unchanged a significant increase in phosphotau is observed in STZ treated mice.

Since phosphorylation state of tau results from a coordinated balance between kinase-mediated phosphorylations of tau and dephosphorylation by protein phosphatases Clodfelder-Miller et al., (Clodfelder-Miller et al., 2006) carried out an extensive assessment of different tau phosphorylation sites and observed accompanied changes in tau kinases, including inhibition of GSK3, by increased phosphorylation on serine-9, as well as increased phosphorylation of both p38 and JNK, indicating activation of these two kinases in mice (Clodfelder-Miller et al., 2006). Also phosphatase PP2A activity, that dephosphorylates multiple residues of tau, was significantly reduced. This study also showed that the whole process, leading to increased tau phosphorylation, is mediated by insulin, since insulin administration after short-term insulin deficiency, provoked by STZ treatment, reduced tau hyperphosphorylation at selective sites (Clodfelder-Miller et al., 2006). The observed changes in phosphatases and kinases, accompanied by the increased phosphorylation of tau on multiple sites, suggested that STZ may impair the natural history of tau, contributing to tau hyperphosphorylation (Clodfelder-Miller et al., 2006). When STZ has been administered to wildtype animals, (Ramos-Rodriguez et al., 2013) a significant increase in tau phosphorylation has also been observed, and although no tangles have been observed, these data support the inductive role of STZ in tau pathology as observed in figure 4.

Although Aβ and tau pathology, as well as neuronal and synaptic loss are the pathological features of AD, cognitive impairment remains the main manifestation of the disease, and following this idea previous studies have also focused on learning and memory alterations associated to peripheral administration of STZ. In this sense it has been well established that STZ-induced diabetes also impaired learning and memory abilities in rodents when tested in different paradigms, including active avoidance tests (Flood et al., 1990, Alvarez et al., 2009) or the Morris water maze test (Ramos-Rodriguez et al., 2013), where significant learning and memory dysfunction has been observed, with altered pathways along the acquisition phase of the test, as observed in figure 5. The close relationship between diabetes and Alzheimer has also been explored in AD mice after STZ treatment, and significantly worse performances in learning and memory processes have been observed (Wang et al., 2010), supporting a synergistic effect between both pathologies. In combination with electrophysiological studies, learning and memory disabilities observed in STZ-treated mice seem to be mediated by alterations in long-term potentiation and depression (Biessels et al., 1996, Artola et al., 2005), whereas hippocampal neurogenesis and synaptic plasticity also seems to be affected (Stranahan et al., 2008). It has also been observed that detected deficits might be recovered after insulin administration, and many other pharmacological approaches have been also shown to have some beneficial effects, including antioxidants such as Ginkgo biloba extract, vitamin E or resveratrol (Hoyer et al., 1999, Tuzcu & Baydas 2006, Schmatz et al., 2009, Comin et al., 2010), non-steroidal anti-inflammatory drugs such as aspirin (Wang et al., 2011) or histone deacetylases ihnibitors such as sodium butyrate (Sharma & Singh 2011).

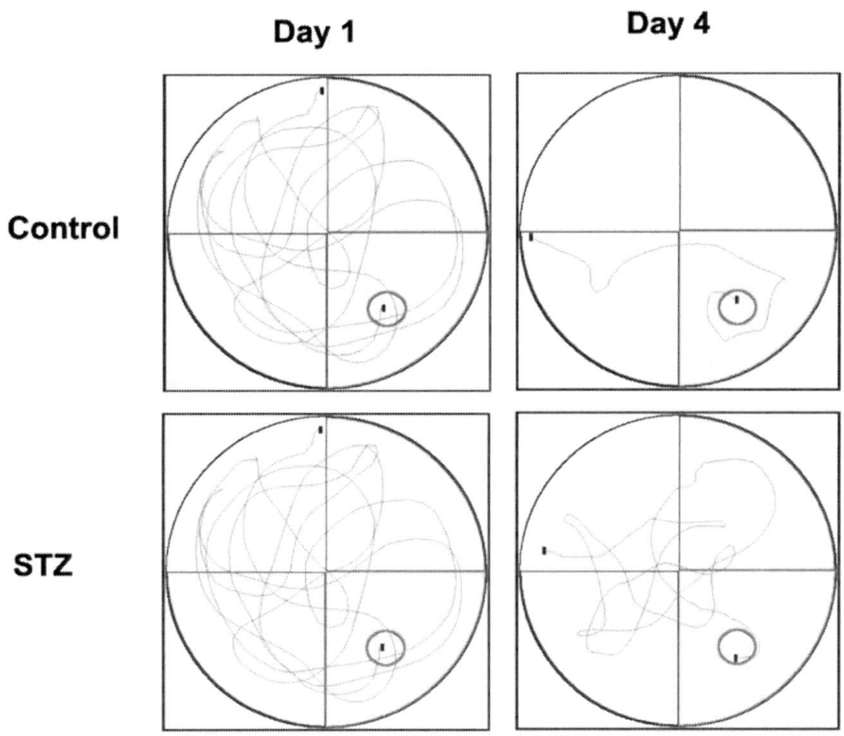


Figure 4. Representative Morris water maze pathways during the first day and the last day of the acquisition phase, both in C57Bl6 control and STZ treated mice (50 mg/Kg ip injection,5 consecutive days). Significantly longer pathways can be observed in STZ treated mice to reach the hidden platform, as an indication of the impairment of these animals to learn and remember the localization of the hidden platform.

## 4.2. Alzheimer´S Disease and Vascular Dementia-Like Complications Associated To Intracerebroventricular Administration of STZ

As shown above, peripheral administration of STZ reproduces or aggravates some of the pathological features observed in AD and VaD, however central delivery of STZ has also been explored, in order to provoke central diabetes, without affecting pancreatic cells.

Intracerebroventricularl (icv) STZ delivering has been used and considered as a model of sporadic AD or T3D, in which it is observed a brain type of non-insulin dependent diabetes, or cerebral diabetes (de la Monte & Wands 2008, Lester-Coll et al., 2006). As previously stated STZ cannot cross the BBB although since GLUT2 receptor are distributed heterogeneously in the mammalian brain, therefore when icv administered, STZ can selectively reduce insulin central levels without affecting insulin and glucose levels in the periphery (Park 2011). Therefore mechanisms, implications and consequences of peripheral or central administration of STZ might be significantly different (Salkovic-Petrisic et al., 2013a). After central STZ administration IGF-1 receptors are reduced, supporting that insulin signaling is impaired in a similar way to that observed in AD patients, where both insulin production and insulin resistance are altered in the brain (Steen et al., 2005, Park 2011). Central STZ administration has been widely used in the last few years, specially in rats, and a recent study systematically compares doses and post-administration end points showing that although at extremely low doses, when compared with peripheral administration, 1mg/kg of STZ icv injected might not be enough to induce cognitive deficits required in the model (Mehla et al., 2013).

Different studies in rodents have shown that local administration of STZ results in central metabolic alterations (Hoyer et al., 1994, Lannert & Hoyer 1998, Labak et al., 2010), including a reduction of glucose utilization in different brain regions (Duelli et al., 1994) or alterations in enzymes implicated in glycolisis and glucogenolysis (Plaschke & Hoyer 1993). Altered glucose metabolism has also been observed, by high-resolution micro-PET 18F-deoxyglucose, in non-human primates after icv infusion of STZ and cortical distribution of glucose hypometabolism seems to resemble that observed at early stages of AD patients (Heo et al., 2011). These authors also detected an increase of sulcal markings by MRI at six weeks post-injection, suggesting brain atrophy, as observed in Alzheimer's patients. Previous studies have also shown neuronal damage and brain atrophy in rodents. In this sense shrinkage of the dorsal hippocampus and adjacent fornix has been observed after icv STZ injections, as well as ventricle enlargement and gliosis in myelinated periventricular brain structures (Weinstock et al., 2001, Shoham et al., 2003). Hippocampal neuronal density has also been observed to be reduced in STZ icv injected rats and it has been suggested that this effect could be mediated by cyclooxygenases 1 and 2 isozymes activity (Dhull et al., 2012). Other STZ studies have also reported septal and white matter atrophy. The basal forebrain, that includes the septum, seems to be a region deeply affected in AD (Teipel et al., 2005) and observed atrophy by MRI was accompanied by a significant reduction of neuronal density in this region, without affecting other brain areas as the striatum (Kraska et al., 2012). Functional manifestation of central alterations have also been observed in icv STZ injected models, and hippocampal synaptic transmission impairment and long-term potentiation alterations have been detected, associated to alterations in integrin-linked kinase-GSK-3-β signaling. This effect may decrease the trafficking and function of postsynaptic glutamate receptors; thereby, leading to synaptic deficits (Shonesy et al., 2010). Other indicative markers of central damage, similar to those also observed in AD patients, have also been detected after icv administration of STZ in rats, including increased oxidative stress and presence of ROS as well as brain reduced antioxidant capacity (Sharma & Gupta 2001, Lester-Coll et al., 2006, Tahirovic et al., 2007).

When tau pathology has been addressed, a significant increase of total tau and phospho tau levels have been observed in the hippocampus of STZ-treated rats (Salkovic-Petrisic et al., 2006, Grunblatt et al., 2007) and similar observations have been made in mice (Chen et al., 2013b), without neurofibrillary tangles deposition. When icv STZ has been administered to a classical AD model as it is the tg2576 mouse, an increase of total tau protein, associated with decreased phosphorylated/total tau ratio has been observed (Plaschke et al., 2010) whereas in 3xTg-AD an increase in tau phosophorylation has been reported (Chen et al., 2013c), suggesting slight differences depending on the animal models and specific experimental approaches used. On the other hand Salkovic-Petrisic et al., have also shown the presence of Aβ aggregates stained with Congo Red both in blood vessels, resembling amyloid angiopathy, and cerebellar plaques in rats icv injected with STZ (Salkovic-Petrisic & Hoyer 2007). This group has recently shown that amyloid angiopathy deposition is observed in wildtype rats up to 9 months after STZ injections, and histological confirmation has included thioflavin S and Congo red staining, as well as in immunohistochemistry studies with anti-Aβ antibodies (Salkovic-Petrisic et al., 2011). Also other studies have shown increased Aβ immunoreactivity in the hippocampus from STZ treated rats (Shingo et al., 2012), as well as increased Aβ levels in different brain regions (Santos et al., 2012) supporting the capacity of the icv STZ model to provoke amyloid pathology, similar to that observed in AD patients. In a transgenic mouse model of AD (tg2576) increased cerebral aggregated Aβ fragments and congophilic amyloid deposits was observed supporting a synergistic effect between icv injected STZ and the overexpression of APP (Plaschke et al., 2010).

Apart from typical neuropathological features associated with AD and VaD, a great deal of attention has been paid to learning and memory alterations observed in icv STZ injected rodents in different paradigms, as well as to the role of therapeutic alternatives to revert observed deficits. In this sense icv injection of STZ in rats results in working and reference memory dysfunction in the holeboard task and the passive avoidance paradigm (Lannert & Hoyer 1998, Salkovic-Petrisic et al., 2013b). Similar alterations have been observed in the delayed non-matching to position task and in working and spatial memory assessed in the Morris water maze test (Prickaerts et al., 1999, Salkovic-Petrisic et al., 2013b), the Y-maze test and novel object recognition tests (Liu et al., 2013). Observed cognition impairment after icv administration of STZ to rats have also been reported in mice, and a worsening effect is observed when STZ is administered to transgenic AD models, such as 3xTg-AD mice (Chen et al., 2013c) or APP overexpressing mice (Plaschke et al., 2010). Since the lack of treatment for AD or VaD remains one of the most relevant issues in the study of the dementia processes, many therapeutic approaches have been used in the icv STZ injected model, and significant improvement of tau phosphorylation and cognitive impairment has been widely observed (for review see (Salkovic-Petrisic et al., 2013a). Following this idea, antioxidant treatments, including resveratrol (Sharma & Gupta 2002), curcumin (Ishrat et al., 2009) or catechin (Ejaz Ahmed et al., 2013) have been shown to improve cognition in STZ treated mice. Also, treatment with statins (Dalla et al., 2010, Tramontina et al., 2011) or ciclooxigenase inhibitors (Dhull et al., 2012) have been shown to recover cognitive impairment associated to icv STZ injection. Moreover presently approved drugs for AD may improve learning and memory dysfunction observed after STZ icv injection, including anticholinesterasic drugs (Sonkusare et al., 2005) and memantine (Ponce-Lopez et al. 2011). The fact that many different pharmacological approaches may help to recover cognitive impairment, and associated central dysfunction after icv STZ administration, supports the multiple and complex pathological pathways affected by STZ, in a similar way to those observed in AD patients.

Altogether, animal models for AD and VaD present evident limitations, and although transgenic mice have proved to be extremely useful to study associated pathology and cognitive impairment, icv injected STZ seems to provide a different approach that resembles biochemical, morphological and cognitive effects associated with an insulin-resistant brain state, similar to that observed in AD patients. On the other hand, since additional treatment options are urgently needed for AD population (for review see (Sabbagh & Cummings 2011) STZ might prove to be a rational animal model in the search of new therapeutic alternatives.

## ACKNOWLEDGMENTS

RYC-2008-02333, ISCIII–Subdirección General de Evaluación y Fomento de la Investigación (PI12/00675) cofinanced by FEDER "Una forma de hacer Europa", Junta de Andalucía, Proyectos de Excelencia (P11-CTS-7847). Thank you to Mr. Juan Jose Ramos Rodriguez for his help with figures included in this chapter.

## REFERENCES

Alvarez, E. O., Beauquis, J., Revsin, Y., Banzan, A. M., Roig, P., De Nicola, A. F. and Saravia, F. (2009) Cognitive dysfunction and hippocampal changes in experimental type 1 diabetes. *Behav Brain Res.* 198, 224-230.

Artola, A., Kamal, A., Ramakers, G. M., Biessels, G. J. and Gispen, W. H. (2005) Diabetes mellitus concomitantly facilitates the induction of long-term depression and inhibits that of long-term potentiation in hippocampus. *Eur. J. Neurosci.* 22, 169-178.

Bhat, N. R. (2010) Linking cardiometabolic disorders to sporadic Alzheimer's disease: a perspective on potential mechanisms and mediators. *J. Neurochem.* 115, 551-562.

Biessels, G. J., Kamal, A., Ramakers, G. M., Urban, I. J., Spruijt, B. M., Erkelens, D. W. and Gispen, W. H. (1996) Place learning and hippocampal synaptic plasticity in streptozotocin-induced diabetic rats. *Diabetes.* 45, 1259-1266.

Brendza, R. P., Bacskai, B. J., Cirrito, J. R. et al. (2005) Anti-Abeta antibody treatment promotes the rapid recovery of amyloid-associated neuritic dystrophy in PDAPP transgenic mice. *J. Clin. Invest.* 115, 428-433.

Brookmeyer, R., Johnson, E., Ziegler-Graham, K. and Arrighi, H. M. (2007) Forecasting the global burden of Alzheimer's disease. *Alzheimers Dement.* 3, 186-191.

Brown, C. E., Aminoltejari, K., Erb, H., Winship, I. R. and Murphy, T. H. (2009) In vivo voltage-sensitive dye imaging in adult mice reveals that somatosensory maps lost to stroke are replaced over weeks by new structural and functional circuits with prolonged modes of activation within both the peri-infarct zone and distant sites. *J. Neurosci.* 29, 1719-1734.

Burke, M. C., Nelson, L., Slade, J. Y., Oakley, A. E., Khundakar, A. A. and Kalaria, R. N. (2013) Morphometry of the hippocampal microvasculature in post-stroke and age-related dementias. *Neuropathol Appl Neurobiol.*

Clodfelder-Miller, B. J., Zmijewska, A. A., Johnson, G. V. and Jope, R. S. (2006) Tau is hyperphosphorylated at multiple sites in mouse brain in vivo after streptozotocin-induced insulin deficiency. *Diabetes*. 55, 3320-3325.

Comin, D., Gazarini, L., Zanoni, J. N., Milani, H. and de Oliveira, R. M. (2010) Vitamin E improves learning performance and changes the expression of nitric oxide-producing neurons in the brains of diabetic rats. *Behav Brain Res*. 210, 38-45.

Correia, S. C., Santos, R. X., Perry, G., Zhu, X., Moreira, P. I. and Smith, M. A. (2011) Insulin-resistant brain state: the culprit in sporadic Alzheimer's disease? *Ageing Res Rev*. 10, 264-273.

Craft, S. (2009) The role of metabolic disorders in Alzheimer disease and vascular dementia: two roads converged. *Arch Neurol*. 66, 300-305.

Craggs, L. J., Hagel, C., Kuhlenbaeumer, G. et al. (2013) Quantitative vascular pathology and phenotyping familial and sporadic cerebral small vessel diseases. *Brain Pathol*. 23, 547-557.

Chen, N., Yang, M., Guo, J., Zhou, M., Zhu, C. and He, L. (2013a) Cerebrolysin for vascular dementia. *Cochrane Database Syst Rev*. 1, CD008900.

Chen, Y., Liang, Z., Blanchard, J. et al. (2013b) A non-transgenic mouse model (icv-STZ mouse) of Alzheimer's disease: similarities to and differences from the transgenic model (3xTg-AD mouse). *Mol. Neurobiol*. 47, 711-725.

Chen, Y., Liang, Z., Tian, Z., Blanchard, J., Dai, C. L., Chalbot, S., Iqbal, K., Liu, F. and Gong, C. X. (2013c) Intracerebroventricular Streptozotocin Exacerbates Alzheimer-Like Changes of 3xTg-AD Mice. *Mol. Neurobiol*.

Dalla, Y., Singh, N., Jaggi, A. S. and Singh, D. (2010) Memory restorative role of statins in experimental dementia: an evidence of their cholesterol dependent and independent actions. *Pharmacol Rep*. 62, 784-796.

de la Monte, S. M. and Wands, J. R. (2008) Alzheimer's disease is type 3 diabetes-evidence reviewed. *J. Diabetes Sci Technol*. 2, 1101-1113.

de Leeuw, F. E., de Groot, J. C., Oudkerk, M., Witteman, J. C., Hofman, A., van Gijn, J. and Breteler, M. M. (2002) Hypertension and cerebral white matter lesions in a prospective cohort study. *Brain*. 125, 765-772.

Devedjian, J. C., George, M., Casellas, A., Pujol, A., Visa, J., Pelegrin, M., Gros, L. and Bosch, F. (2000) Transgenic mice overexpressing insulin-like growth factor-II in beta cells develop type 2 diabetes. *J. Clin. Invest*. 105, 731-740.

Devi, L., Alldred, M. J., Ginsberg, S. D. and Ohno, M. (2012) Mechanisms underlying insulin deficiency-induced acceleration of beta-amyloidosis in a mouse model of Alzheimer's disease. *PLoS One*. 7, e32792.

Dhull, D. K., Bhateja, D., Dhull, R. K. and Padi, S. S. (2012) Differential role of cyclooxygenase isozymes on neuronal density in hippocampus CA1 region of intracerebroventricular streptozotocin treated rat brain. *J. Chem. Neuroanat*. 43, 48-51.

Ding, Y., Zhang, Z., Dai, X., Jiang, Y., Bao, L. and Li, Y. (2013) Grape seed proanthocyanidins ameliorate pancreatic beta-cell dysfunction and death in low-dose streptozotocin- and high-carbohydrate/high-fat diet-induced diabetic rats partially by regulating endoplasmic reticulum stress. *Nutr. Metab* (Lond). 10, 51.

Duelli, R., Schrock, H., Kuschinsky, W. and Hoyer, S. (1994) Intracerebroventricular injection of streptozotocin induces discrete local changes in cerebral glucose utilization in rats. *Int. J. Dev. Neurosci*. 12, 737-743.

Dumont, M. and Beal, M. F. (2011) Neuroprotective strategies involving ROS in Alzheimer disease. *Free Radic Biol. Med.* 51, 1014-1026.

Eckman, E. A. and Eckman, C. B. (2005) Abeta-degrading enzymes: modulators of Alzheimer's disease pathogenesis and targets for therapeutic intervention. *Biochem. Soc Trans.* 33, 1101-1105.

Ejaz Ahmed, M., Khan, M. M., Javed, H., Vaibhav, K., Khan, A., Tabassum, R., Ashafaq, M., Islam, F. and Safhi, M. M. (2013) Amelioration of cognitive impairment and neurodegeneration by catechin hydrate in rat model of streptozotocin-induced experimental dementia of Alzheimer's type. *Neurochem Int.* 62, 492-501.

Farris, W., Mansourian, S., Chang, Y. et al. (2003) Insulin-degrading enzyme regulates the levels of insulin, amyloid beta-protein, and the beta-amyloid precursor protein intracellular domain in vivo. *Proc. Natl. Acad. Sci. USA.* 100, 4162-4167.

Flood, J. F., Mooradian, A. D. and Morley, J. E. (1990) Characteristics of learning and memory in streptozocin-induced diabetic mice. *Diabetes.* 39, 1391-1398.

Frisoni, G. B., Fox, N. C., Jack, C. R., Jr., Scheltens, P. and Thompson, P. M. (2010) The clinical use of structural MRI in Alzheimer disease. *Nat. Rev Neurol.* 6, 67-77.

Frolich, L., Blum-Degen, D., Bernstein, H. G. et al. (1998) Brain insulin and insulin receptors in aging and sporadic Alzheimer's disease. *J. Neural Transm.* 105, 423-438.

Frydman-Marom, A., Levin, A., Farfara, D. et al. (2011) Orally administrated cinnamon extract reduces beta-amyloid oligomerization and corrects cognitive impairment in Alzheimer's disease animal models. *PLoS One.* 6, e16564.

Garcia-Alloza, M., Borrelli, L. A., Hyman, B. T. and Bacskai, B. J. (2010) Antioxidants have a rapid and long-lasting effect on neuritic abnormalities in APP:PS1 mice. *Neurobiol Aging.* 31, 2058-2068.

Garcia-Alloza, M., Dodwell, S. A., Meyer-Luehmann, M., Hyman, B. T. and Bacskai, B. J. (2006a) Plaque-derived oxidative stress mediates distorted neurite trajectories in the Alzheimer mouse model. *J. Neuropathol Exp. Neurol.* 65, 1082-1089.

Garcia-Alloza, M., Prada, C., Lattarulo, C., Fine, S., Borrelli, L. A., Betensky, R., Greenberg, S. M., Frosch, M. P. and Bacskai, B. J. (2009) Matrix metalloproteinase inhibition reduces oxidative stress associated with cerebral amyloid angiopathy in vivo in transgenic mice. *J. Neurochem. 109*, 1636-1647.

Garcia-Alloza, M., Robbins, E. M., Zhang-Nunes, S. X. et al. (2006b) Characterization of amyloid deposition in the APPswe/PS1dE9 mouse model of Alzheimer disease. *Neurobiol. Dis.* 24, 516-524.

Gomez-Isla, T., Hollister, R., West, H., Mui, S., Growdon, J. H., Petersen, R. C., Parisi, J. E. and Hyman, B. T. (1997) Neuronal loss correlates with but exceeds neurofibrillary tangles in Alzheimer's disease. *Ann. Neurol.* 41, 17-24.

Gong, C. X., Grundke-Iqbal, I. and Iqbal, K. (2010) Targeting tau protein in Alzheimer's disease. *Drugs Aging.* 27, 351-365.

Gorelick, P. B. (2004) Risk factors for vascular dementia and Alzheimer disease. *Stroke.* 35, 2620-2622.

Gorelick, P. B. and Nyenhuis, D. (2013) Understanding and treating vascular cognitive impairment. *Continuum* (Minneap Minn). 19, 425-437.

Gotz, J., Ittner, L. M. and Lim, Y. A. (2009) Common features between diabetes mellitus and Alzheimer's disease. *Cell Mol Life Sci.* 66, 1321-1325.

Greenberg, S. M., Grabowski, T., Gurol, M. E. et al. (2008) Detection of isolated cerebrovascular beta-amyloid with Pittsburgh compound B. *Ann Neurol*. 64, 587-591.

Grunblatt, E., Salkovic-Petrisic, M., Osmanovic, J., Riederer, P. and Hoyer, S. (2007) Brain insulin system dysfunction in streptozotocin intracerebroventricularly treated rats generates hyperphosphorylated tau protein. *J. Neurochem*. 101, 757-770.

Guglielmotto, M., Aragno, M., Tamagno, E. et al. (2012) AGEs/RAGE complex upregulates BACE1 via NF-kappaB pathway activation. *Neurobiol Aging*. 33, 196 e113-127.

Harman, D. (2006) Alzheimer's disease pathogenesis: role of aging. *Ann N Y Acad Sci*. 1067, 454-460.

He, Y., Zheng, M. M., Ma, Y., Han, X. J., Ma, X. Q., Qu, C. Q. and Du, Y. F. (2013) Soluble oligomers and fibrillar species of amyloid beta-peptide differentially affect cognitive functions and hippocampal inflammatory response. *Biochem Biophys Res Commun*. 429, 125-130.

Heo, J. H., Lee, S. R., Lee, S. T., Lee, K. M., Oh, J. H., Jang, D. P., Chang, K. T. and Cho, Z. H. (2011) Spatial distribution of glucose hypometabolism induced by intracerebroventricular streptozotocin in monkeys. *J. Alzheimers Dis*. 25, 517-523.

Hiltunen, M., Khandelwal, V. K., Yaluri, N. et al. (2012) Contribution of genetic and dietary insulin resistance to Alzheimer phenotype in APP/PS1 transgenic mice. *J. Cell Mol Med*. 16, 1206-1222.

Honig, L. S., Kukull, W. and Mayeux, R. (2005) Atherosclerosis and AD: analysis of data from the US National Alzheimer's Coordinating Center. *Neurology*. 64, 494-500.

Hoyer, S., Lannert, H., Noldner, M. and Chatterjee, S. S. (1999) Damaged neuronal energy metabolism and behavior are improved by Ginkgo biloba extract (EGb 761). *J. Neural Transm*. 106, 1171-1188.

Hoyer, S., Muller, D. and Plaschke, K. (1994) Desensitization of brain insulin receptor. Effect on glucose/energy and related metabolism. *J. Neural Transm Suppl*. 44, 259-268.

Hyman, B. T. (2011) Amyloid-dependent and amyloid-independent stages of Alzheimer disease. *Arch. Neurol*. 68, 1062-1064.

Hyman, B. T. and Gomez-Isla, T. (1996) Neuropathological markers of impaired cognition in the entorhinal cortex. *Neurobiol Aging*. 17, 940-941; discussion 945-947.

Hyman, B. T. and Trojanowski, J. Q. (1997) Consensus recommendations for the postmortem diagnosis of Alzheimer disease from the National Institute on Aging and the Reagan Institute Working Group on diagnostic criteria for the neuropathological assessment of Alzheimer disease. J Neuropathol Exp Neurol. 56, 1095-1097.

Ishrat, T., Hoda, M. N., Khan, M. B., Yousuf, S., Ahmad, M., Khan, M. M., Ahmad, A. and Islam, F. (2009) Amelioration of cognitive deficits and neurodegeneration by curcumin in rat model of sporadic dementia of Alzheimer's type (SDAT). *Eur Neuropsychopharmacol*. 19, 636-647.

Ivan, C. S., Seshadri, S., Beiser, A., Au, R., Kase, C. S., Kelly-Hayes, M. and Wolf, P. A. (2004) Dementia after stroke: the Framingham Study. *Stroke*. 35, 1264-1268.

Jankowsky, J. L., Fadale, D. J., Anderson, J. et al. (2004) Mutant presenilins specifically elevate the levels of the 42 residue beta-amyloid peptide in vivo: evidence for augmentation of a 42-specific gamma secretase. *Hum Mol Genet*. 13, 159-170.

Jelinek, D., Millward, V., Birdi, A., Trouard, T. P., Heidenreich, R. A. and Garver, W. S. (2011) Npc1 haploinsufficiency promotes weight gain and metabolic features associated with insulin resistance. *Hum. Mol Genet*. 20, 312-321.

Jimenez-Palomares, M., Ramos-Rodriguez, J. J., Lopez-Acosta, J. F., Pacheco-Herrero, M., Lechuga-Sancho, A. M., Perdomo, G., Garcia-Alloza, M. and Cozar-Castellano, I. (2012) Increased Abeta production prompts the onset of glucose intolerance and insulin resistance. *Am. J. Physiol Endocrinol Metab*. 302, E1373-1380.

Jolivalt, C. G., Calcutt, N. A. and Masliah, E. (2012) Similar pattern of peripheral neuropathy in mouse models of type 1 diabetes and Alzheimer's disease. *Neuroscience*. 202, 405-412.

Jolivalt, C. G., Hurford, R., Lee, C. A., Dumaop, W., Rockenstein, E. and Masliah, E. (2010) Type 1 diabetes exaggerates features of Alzheimer's disease in APP transgenic mice. *Exp. Neurol.* 223, 422-431.

Jolivalt, C. G., Lee, C. A., Beiswenger, K. K., Smith, J. L., Orlov, M., Torrance, M. A. and Masliah, E. (2008) Defective insulin signaling pathway and increased glycogen synthase kinase-3 activity in the brain of diabetic mice: parallels with Alzheimer's disease and correction by insulin. *J. Neurosci Res.* 86, 3265-3274.

Ke, Y. D., Delerue, F., Gladbach, A., Gotz, J. and Ittner, L. M. (2009) Experimental diabetes mellitus exacerbates tau pathology in a transgenic mouse model of Alzheimer's disease. *PLoS One*. 4, e7917.

Knowles, R. B., Wyart, C., Buldyrev, S. V., Cruz, L., Urbanc, B., Hasselmo, M. E., Stanley, H. E. and Hyman, B. T. (1999) Plaque-induced neurite abnormalities: implications for disruption of neural networks in Alzheimer's disease. *Proc. Natl. Acad. Sci. USA*. 96, 5274-5279.

Konarkowska, B., Aitken, J. F., Kistler, J., Zhang, S. and Cooper, G. J. (2006) The aggregation potential of human amylin determines its cytotoxicity towards islet beta-cells. *Febs J.* 273, 3614-3624.

Kraska, A., Santin, M. D., Dorieux, O. et al. (2012) In vivo cross-sectional characterization of cerebral alterations induced by intracerebroventricular administration of streptozotocin. *PLoS One*. 7, e46196.

Labak, M., Foniok, T., Kirk, D., Rushforth, D., Tomanek, B., Jasinski, A. and Grieb, P. (2010) Metabolic changes in rat brain following intracerebroventricular injections of streptozotocin: a model of sporadic Alzheimer's disease. *Acta Neurochir Suppl.* 106, 177-181.

Lannert, H. and Hoyer, S. (1998) Intracerebroventricular administration of streptozotocin causes long-term diminutions in learning and memory abilities and in cerebral energy metabolism in adult rats. *Behav. Neurosci.* 112, 1199-1208.

Larson, J., Lynch, G., Games, D. and Seubert, P. (1999) Alterations in synaptic transmission and long-term potentiation in hippocampal slices from young and aged PDAPP mice. *Brain Res.* 840, 23-35.

Lee, M. S. (2013) Treatment of Autoimmune Diabetes by Inhibiting the Initial Event. *Immune Netw*. 13, 194-198.

Lester-Coll, N., Rivera, E. J., Soscia, S. J., Doiron, K., Wands, J. R. and de la Monte, S. M. (2006) Intracerebral streptozotocin model of type 3 diabetes: relevance to sporadic Alzheimer's disease. *J. Alzheimers Dis.* 9, 13-33.

Li, Y., Duffy, K. B., Ottinger, M. A. et al. (2010) GLP-1 receptor stimulation reduces amyloid-beta peptide accumulation and cytotoxicity in cellular and animal models of Alzheimer's disease. *J. Alzheimers Dis.* 19, 1205-1219.

Liu, P., Zou, L. B., Wang, L. H., Jiao, Q., Chi, T. Y., Ji, X. F. and Jin, G. (2013) Xanthoceraside attenuates tau hyperphosphorylation and cognitive deficits in intracerebroventricular-streptozotocin injected rats. *Psychopharmacology* (Berl).

Lombardo, J. A., Stern, E. A., McLellan, M. E., Kajdasz, S. T., Hickey, G. A., Bacskai, B. J. and Hyman, B. T. (2003) Amyloid-beta antibody treatment leads to rapid normalization of plaque-induced neuritic alterations. *J. Neurosci.* 23, 10879-10883.

Luchsinger, J. A., Reitz, C., Honig, L. S., Tang, M. X., Shea, S. and Mayeux, R. (2005) Aggregation of vascular risk factors and risk of incident Alzheimer disease. *Neurology.* 65, 545-551.

Luchsinger, J. A., Tang, M. X., Shea, S. and Mayeux, R. (2004) Hyperinsulinemia and risk of Alzheimer disease. *Neurology*. 63, 1187-1192.

Matsuzaki, T., Sasaki, K., Tanizaki, Y. et al. (2010) Insulin resistance is associated with the pathology of Alzheimer disease: the Hisayama study. *Neurology*. 75, 764-770.

Matveyenko, A. V. and Butler, P. C. (2006) Beta-cell deficit due to increased apoptosis in the human islet amyloid polypeptide transgenic (HIP) rat recapitulates the metabolic defects present in type 2 diabetes. *Diabetes.* 55, 2106-2114.

Mehla, J., Pahuja, M. and Gupta, Y. K. (2013) Streptozotocin-induced sporadic Alzheimer's disease: selection of appropriate dose. *J. Alzheimers Dis*. 33, 17-21.

Meyer-Luehmann, M., Spires-Jones, T. L., Prada, C. et al. (2008) Rapid appearance and local toxicity of amyloid-beta plaques in a mouse model of Alzheimer's disease. *Nature.* 451, 720-724.

Moorhouse, P. and Rockwood, K. (2008) Vascular cognitive impairment: current concepts and clinical developments. *Lancet Neurol.* 7, 246-255.

Mukai, N., Hori, S. and Pomeroy, M. (1980) Cerebral lesions in rats with streptozotocin-induced diabetes. *Acta Neuropathol.* 51, 79-84.

Nugent, D. A., Smith, D. M. and Jones, H. B. (2008) A review of islet of Langerhans degeneration in rodent models of type 2 diabetes. *Toxicol Pathol*. 36, 529-551.

O'Brien, J. T. (2006) Vascular cognitive impairment. *Am. J. Geriatr Psychiatry*. 14, 724-733.

Orgogozo, J. M., Gilman, S., Dartigues, J. F. et al. (2003) Subacute meningoencephalitis in a subset of patients with AD after Abeta42 immunization. *Neurology.* 61, 46-54.

Ott, A., Stolk, R. P., Hofman, A., van Harskamp, F., Grobbee, D. E. and Breteler, M. M. (1996) Association of diabetes mellitus and dementia: the Rotterdam Study. *Diabetologia.* 39, 1392-1397.

Pappolla, M. A. (2008) Statins, incident Alzheimer disease, change in cognitive function, and neuropathology. *Neurology*. 71, 2020; author reply 2020-2021.

Pappolla, M. A., Bryant-Thomas, T. K., Herbert, D. et al. (2003) Mild hypercholesterolemia is an early risk factor for the development of Alzheimer amyloid pathology. Neurology. 61, 199-205.

Park, S. A. (2011) A common pathogenic mechanism linking type-2 diabetes and Alzheimer's disease: evidence from animal models. *J. Clin. Neurol.* 7, 10-18.

Patel, B. M. and Bhadada, S. V. (2013) Type 2 diabetes-induced cardiovascular complications: comparative evaluation of spironolactone, atenolol, metoprolol, ramipril and perindopril. *Clin. Exp. Hypertens*.

Plaschke, K. and Hoyer, S. (1993) Action of the diabetogenic drug streptozotocin on glycolytic and glycogenolytic metabolism in adult rat brain cortex and hippocampus. *Int. J. Dev. Neurosci*. 11, 477-483.

Plaschke, K., Kopitz, J., Siegelin, M., Schliebs, R., Salkovic-Petrisic, M., Riederer, P. and Hoyer, S. (2010) Insulin-resistant brain state after intracerebroventricular streptozotocin injection exacerbates Alzheimer-like changes in Tg2576 AbetaPP-overexpressing mice. *J. Alzheimers Dis.* 19, 691-704.

Plastino, M., Fava, A., Pirritano, D. et al. (2010) Effects of insulinic therapy on cognitive impairment in patients with Alzheimer disease and diabetes mellitus type-2. *J. Neurol Sci.* 288, 112-116.

Ponce-Lopez, T., Liy-Salmeron, G., Hong, E. and Meneses, A. (2011) Lithium, phenserine, memantine and pioglitazone reverse memory deficit and restore phospho-GSK3beta decreased in hippocampus in intracerebroventricular streptozotocin induced memory deficit model. *Brain Res.* 1426, 73-85.

Prickaerts, J., Fahrig, T. and Blokland, A. (1999) Cognitive performance and biochemical markers in septum, hippocampus and striatum of rats after an i.c.v. injection of streptozotocin: a correlation analysis. *Behav. Brain Res.* 102, 73-88.

Qiu, W. Q., Walsh, D. M., Ye, Z. et al. (1998) Insulin-degrading enzyme regulates extracellular levels of amyloid beta-protein by degradation. *J. Biol. Chem.* 273, 32730-32738.

Ramos-Rodriguez, J. J., Ortiz, O., Jimenez-Palomares, M. et al. (2013) Differential central pathology and cognitive impairment in pre-diabetic and diabetic mice. *Psychoneuroendocrinology.* 38, 2462-2475.

Reitz, C., Tang, M. X., Manly, J., Mayeux, R. and Luchsinger, J. A. (2007) Hypertension and the risk of mild cognitive impairment. *Arch. Neurol.* 64, 1734-1740.

Revsin, Y., Rekers, N. V., Louwe, M. C., Saravia, F. E., De Nicola, A. F., de Kloet, E. R. and Oitzl, M. S. (2009) Glucocorticoid receptor blockade normalizes hippocampal alterations and cognitive impairment in streptozotocin-induced type 1 diabetes mice. *Neuropsychopharmacology.* 34, 747-758.

Roberson, M. R. and Harrell, L. E. (1997) Cholinergic activity and amyloid precursor protein metabolism. *Brain Res. Brain Res. Rev.* 25, 50-69.

Roman, G. C. (2005) Vascular dementia prevention: a risk factor analysis. *Cerebrovasc Dis.* 20 Suppl 2, 91-100.

Russell, J. C. and Proctor, S. D. (2006) Small animal models of cardiovascular disease: tools for the study of the roles of metabolic syndrome, dyslipidemia, and atherosclerosis. *Cardiovasc. Pathol.* 15, 318-330.

Sabbagh, M. and Cummings, J. (2011) Progressive cholinergic decline in Alzheimer's Disease: consideration for treatment with donepezil 23 mg in patients with moderate to severe symptomatology. *BMC Neurol.* 11, 21.

Salkovic-Petrisic, M. and Hoyer, S. (2007) Central insulin resistance as a trigger for sporadic Alzheimer-like pathology: an experimental approach. *J. Neural Transm Suppl.* 217-233.

Salkovic-Petrisic, M., Knezovic, A., Hoyer, S. and Riederer, P. (2013a) What have we learned from the streptozotocin-induced animal model of sporadic Alzheimer's disease, about the therapeutic strategies in Alzheimer's research. *J. Neural Transm.* 120, 233-252.

Salkovic-Petrisic, M., Osmanovic-Barilar, J., Bruckner, M. K., Hoyer, S., Arendt, T. and Riederer, P. (2011) Cerebral amyloid angiopathy in streptozotocin rat model of sporadic Alzheimer's disease: a long-term follow up study. *J. Neural Transm.* 118, 765-772.

Salkovic-Petrisic, M., Osmanovic-Barilar, J., Knezovic, A., Hoyer, S., Mosetter, K. and Reutter, W. (2013b) Long-term oral galactose treatment prevents cognitive deficits in male Wistar rats treated intracerebroventricularly with streptozotocin. *Neuropharmacology.* 77C, 68-80.

Salkovic-Petrisic, M., Tribl, F., Schmidt, M., Hoyer, S. and Riederer, P. (2006) Alzheimer-like changes in protein kinase B and glycogen synthase kinase-3 in rat frontal cortex and hippocampus after damage to the insulin signalling pathway. *J. Neurochem.* 96, 1005-1015.

Santos, T. O., Mazucanti, C. H., Xavier, G. F. and Torrao, A. S. (2012) Early and late neurodegeneration and memory disruption after intracerebroventricular streptozotocin. *Physiol Behav.* 107, 401-413.

Saxena, R., Voight, B. F., Lyssenko, V. et al. (2007) Genome-wide association analysis identifies loci for type 2 diabetes and triglyceride levels. *Science.* 316, 1331-1336.

Schliebs, R. and Arendt, T. (2006) The significance of the cholinergic system in the brain during aging and in Alzheimer's disease. *J. Neural Transm.* 113, 1625-1644.

Schmatz, R., Mazzanti, C. M., Spanevello, R. et al. (2009) Resveratrol prevents memory deficits and the increase in acetylcholinesterase activity in streptozotocin-induced diabetic rats. *Eur. J. Pharmacol.* 610, 42-48.

Schrijvers, E. M., Witteman, J. C., Sijbrands, E. J., Hofman, A., Koudstaal, P. J. and Breteler, M. M. (2010) Insulin metabolism and the risk of Alzheimer disease: the Rotterdam Study. *Neurology*. 75, 1982-1987.

Serrano-Pozo, A., Frosch, M. P., Masliah, E. and Hyman, B. T. (2011) Neuropathological alterations in Alzheimer disease. *Cold Spring Harb Perspect Med.* 1, a006189.

Seshadri, S., Beiser, A., Selhub, J., Jacques, P. F., Rosenberg, I. H., D'Agostino, R. B., Wilson, P. W. and Wolf, P. A. (2002) Plasma homocysteine as a risk factor for dementia and Alzheimer's disease. *N Engl J Med.* 346, 476-483.

Sharma, B. and Singh, N. (2010) Pitavastatin and 4'-hydroxy-3'-methoxyacetophenone (HMAP) reduce cognitive dysfunction in vascular dementia during experimental diabetes. Curr Neurovasc Res. 7, 180-191.

Sharma, B. and Singh, N. (2011) Attenuation of vascular dementia by sodium butyrate in streptozotocin diabetic rats. *Psychopharmacology* (Berl). 215, 677-687.

Sharma, M. and Gupta, Y. K. (2001) Intracerebroventricular injection of streptozotocin in rats produces both oxidative stress in the brain and cognitive impairment. *Life Sci.* 68, 1021-1029.

Sharma, M. and Gupta, Y. K. (2002) Chronic treatment with trans resveratrol prevents intracerebroventricular streptozotocin induced cognitive impairment and oxidative stress in rats. *Life Sci.* 71, 2489-2498.

Shingo, A. S., Kanabayashi, T., Murase, T. and Kito, S. (2012) Cognitive decline in STZ-3V rats is largely due to dysfunctional insulin signalling through the dentate gyrus. *Behav Brain Res.* 229, 378-383.

Shoham, S., Bejar, C., Kovalev, E. and Weinstock, M. (2003) Intracerebroventricular injection of streptozotocin causes neurotoxicity to myelin that contributes to spatial memory deficits in rats. *Exp Neurol.* 184, 1043-1052.

Shonesy, B. C., Thiruchelvam, K., Parameshwaran, K. et al. (2010) Central insulin resistance and synaptic dysfunction in intracerebroventricular-streptozotocin injected rodents. *Neurobiol Aging.* 33, 430 e435-418.

Sonkusare, S., Srinivasan, K., Kaul, C. and Ramarao, P. (2005) Effect of donepezil and lercanidipine on memory impairment induced by intracerebroventricular streptozotocin in rats. *Life Sci.* 77, 1-14.

Spires, T. L., Meyer-Luehmann, M., Stern, E. A., McLean, P. J., Skoch, J., Nguyen, P. T., Bacskai, B. J. and Hyman, B. T. (2005) Dendritic spine abnormalities in amyloid precursor protein transgenic mice demonstrated by gene transfer and intravital multiphoton microscopy. *J Neurosci.* 25, 7278-7287.

Srinivasan, K., Viswanad, B., Asrat, L., Kaul, C. L. and Ramarao, P. (2005) Combination of high-fat diet-fed and low-dose streptozotocin-treated rat: a model for type 2 diabetes and pharmacological screening. *Pharmacol Res.* 52, 313-320.

Steen, E., Terry, B. M., Rivera, E. J., Cannon, J. L., Neely, T. R., Tavares, R., Xu, X. J., Wands, J. R. and de la Monte, S. M. (2005) Impaired insulin and insulin-like growth factor expression and signaling mechanisms in Alzheimer's disease--is this type 3 diabetes? *J. Alzheimers Dis.* 7, 63-80.

Stern, E. A., Bacskai, B. J., Hickey, G. A., Attenello, F. J., Lombardo, J. A. and Hyman, B. T. (2004) Cortical synaptic integration in vivo is disrupted by amyloid-beta plaques. *J. Neurosci.* 24, 4535-4540.

Strachan, M. W., Reynolds, R. M., Frier, B. M., Mitchell, R. J. and Price, J. F. (2008) The relationship between type 2 diabetes and dementia. *Br. Med. Bull.* 88, 131-146.

Stranahan, A. M., Arumugam, T. V., Cutler, R. G., Lee, K., Egan, J. M. and Mattson, M. P. (2008) Diabetes impairs hippocampal function through glucocorticoid-mediated effects on new and mature neurons. *Nat. Neurosci.* 11, 309-317.

Tahirovic, I., Sofic, E., Sapcanin, A., Gavrankapetanovic, I., Bach-Rojecky, L., Salkovic-Petrisic, M., Lackovic, Z., Hoyer, S. and Riederer, P. (2007) Reduced brain antioxidant capacity in rat models of betacytotoxic-induced experimental sporadic Alzheimer's disease and diabetes mellitus. *Neurochem. Res.* 32, 1709-1717.

Takeda, S., Sato, N., Uchio-Yamada, K. et al. (2010) Diabetes-accelerated memory dysfunction via cerebrovascular inflammation and Abeta deposition in an Alzheimer mouse model with diabetes. *Proc. Natl. Acad. Sci. USA*. 107, 7036-7041.

Teipel, S. J., Flatz, W. H., Heinsen, H. et al. (2005) Measurement of basal forebrain atrophy in Alzheimer's disease using MRI. *Brain*. 128, 2626-2644.

Tramontina, A. C., Wartchow, K. M., Rodrigues, L., Biasibetti, R., Quincozes-Santos, A., Bobermin, L., Tramontina, F. and Goncalves, C. A. (2011) The neuroprotective effect of two statins: simvastatin and pravastatin on a streptozotocin-induced model of Alzheimer's disease in rats. *J. Neural Transm.* 118, 1641-1649.

Tuzcu, M. and Baydas, G. (2006) Effect of melatonin and vitamin E on diabetes-induced learning and memory impairment in rats. *Eur. J. Pharmacol.* 537, 106-110.

Urbanc, B., Cruz, L., Le, R., Sanders, J., Ashe, K. H., Duff, K., Stanley, H. E., Irizarry, M. C. and Hyman, B. T. (2002) Neurotoxic effects of thioflavin S-positive amyloid deposits in transgenic mice and Alzheimer's disease. *Proc. Natl. Acad. Sci. USA*. 99, 13990-13995.

Vekrellis, K., Ye, Z., Qiu, W. Q., Walsh, D., Hartley, D., Chesneau, V., Rosner, M. R. and Selkoe, D. J. (2000) Neurons regulate extracellular levels of amyloid beta-protein via proteolysis by insulin-degrading enzyme. J. Neurosci. 20, 1657-1665.

Walsh, D. M. and Selkoe, D. J. (2004) Deciphering the molecular basis of memory failure in Alzheimer's disease. *Neuron*. 44, 181-193.

Wang, T., Fu, F. H., Han, B., Zhang, L. M. and Zhang, X. M. (2011) Long-term but not short-term aspirin treatment attenuates diabetes-associated learning and memory decline in mice. *Exp. Clin. Endocrinol Diabetes*. 119, 36-40.

Wang, X., Zheng, W., Xie, J. W., Wang, T., Wang, S. L., Teng, W. P. and Wang, Z. Y. (2010) Insulin deficiency exacerbates cerebral amyloidosis and behavioral deficits in an Alzheimer transgenic mouse model. *Mol. Neurodegener*. 5, 46.

Weedon, M. N. and Frayling, T. M. (2007) Insights on pathogenesis of type 2 diabetes from MODY genetics. *Curr. Diab. Rep*. 7, 131-138.

Weinstock, M., Kirschbaum-Slager, N., Lazarovici, P., Bejar, C., Youdim, M. B. and Shoham, S. (2001) Neuroprotective effects of novel cholinesterase inhibitors derived from rasagiline as potential anti-Alzheimer drugs. *Ann. N Y Acad Sci*. 939, 148-161.

Wild, S., Roglic, G., Green, A., Sicree, R. and King, H. (2004) Global prevalence of diabetes: estimates for the year 2000 and projections for 2030. *Diabetes Care*. 27, 1047-1053.

Wimo, A., Jonsson, L. and Winblad, B. (2006) An estimate of the worldwide prevalence and direct costs of dementia in 2003. *Dement Geriatr Cogn Disord*. 21, 175-181.

Woodhouse, A., West, A. K., Chuckowree, J. A., Vickers, J. C. and Dickson, T. C. (2005) Does beta-amyloid plaque formation cause structural injury to neuronal processes? *Neurotox Res*. 7, 5-15.

Yang, Y., Ma, D., Wang, Y., Jiang, T., Hu, S., Zhang, M., Yu, X. and Gong, C. X. (2013a) Intranasal insulin ameliorates tau hyperphosphorylation in a rat model of type 2 diabetes. *J. Alzheimers Dis*. 33, 329-338.

Yang, Y., Zhang, J., Ma, D., Zhang, M., Hu, S., Shao, S. and Gong, C. X. (2013b) Subcutaneous administration of liraglutide ameliorates Alzheimer-associated tau hyperphosphorylation in rats with type 2 diabetes. *J. Alzheimers Dis*. 37, 637-648.

Yao, J., Du, H., Yan, S. et al. (2011) Inhibition of amyloid-beta (Abeta) peptide-binding alcohol dehydrogenase-Abeta interaction reduces Abeta accumulation and improves mitochondrial function in a mouse model of Alzheimer's disease. *J. Neurosci*. 31, 2313-2320.

Zhang, M., Lv, X. Y., Li, J., Xu, Z. G. and Chen, L. (2008) The characterization of high-fat diet and multiple low-dose streptozotocin induced type 2 diabetes rat model. *Exp. Diabetes Res*. 2008, 704045.

Zhang, S. and Murphy, T. H. (2007) Imaging the impact of cortical microcirculation on synaptic structure and sensory-evoked hemodynamic responses in vivo. *PLoS Biol*. 5, e119.

Zhao, W. Q., De Felice, F. G., Fernandez, S., Chen, H., Lambert, M. P., Quon, M. J., Krafft, G. A. and Klein, W. L. (2008) Amyloid beta oligomers induce impairment of neuronal insulin receptors. *Faseb J*. 22, 246-260.

In: Streptozotocin: Uses, Mechanism of Action and Side Effects ISBN: 978-1-63117-255-7
Editor: Elizabeth L. Gauthier 

*Chapter 2*

# USE OF STREPTOZOTOCIN IN EXPERIMENTAL TYPE 1 DIABETIC MODELS

***Jing Zhang[1,2,3] and Laura R. McCabe[3,*]***

[1]Bone and Joint Research Center, First affiliated hospital of Xi'an Jiaotong University, Xi'an, Shaanxi, People's Republic of China

[2]Frontier Institute of Science and Technology, Xi'an Jiaotong University, Xi'an, Shaanxi, People's Republic of China

[3]Departments of Physiology and Radiology, Michigan State University, East Lansing, MI, US

## ABSTRACT

Streptozotocin (STZ), an antibiotic and anticancer agent, is the most prominent diabetogenic chemical agent in diabetes research due to its cytotoxicity to the pancreatic beta-cells. The selective toxicity of STZ to beta cells occurs because of its preferential accumulation in beta cells through uptake via GLUT2 glucose transporter. Insulin dependent diabetes mellitus can be induced by either single high dose or multiple low-dose STZ injections. At low dose, STZ induces pancreatic beta-cell apoptosis and at high dose it causes necrosis. The methylnitrosourea moiety derived from STZ has alkylating properties and is thought to modify macromolecules and break DNA strands which depletes the intracellular $NAD^+$ levels and inhibits beta cell function and insulin secretion. STZ also provokes oxidative stress that further contributes to beta cell toxicity. Though STZ itself can cause carcinogenesis and renal, hepatic and muscle myoblast toxicity, these side effects can be minimized or completely avoided by using lower doses. In addition, changes observed weeks after diabetes induction are less likely to result from direct effects of STZ as confirmed in spontaneous diabetic models. For example, multiple low-dose STZ induced diabetic rodent models display bone loss and show similar body parameters changes as spontaneous diabetic mouse models and diabetic patients. It is for this reason that STZ has been wildly used and serves as useful tools to examine mechanisms of type 1 diabetes and its complications.

* Editorial correspondence and reprint requests to: Laura R. McCabe, Ph.D.; Michigan State University, Departments of Physiology and Radiology, 2201 Biomedical Physical Science Bldg., East Lansing, MI 48824; (517) 884-5152; (517) 355-5125 Fax: mccabel@msu.edu. Authors have nothing to disclose.

## INTRODUCTION

Diabetes is reaching epidemic proportions in developed countries. Type 1 diabetes, the most common form of newly diagnosed diabetes in childhood [1], afflicts both males and females at all stages of life [2-4]. To determine the pathology of type 1 diabetes and search for novel antidiabetic agents, a number of diabetic animal models have been developed and improved over the years, of which rodent models are the most thoroughly described. These models can be classified into two broad categories: 1) genetically induced spontaneous diabetes models; and 2) pharmacologicallly induced nonspontaneous diabetes models. Comparatively lower cost, ease of diabetes induction, ease of maintenance, higher rate of animals with typical phenotypes and wider availability make the pharmacologically induced nonspontaneous models more popular in diabetes research than the genetically induced spontaneous models. Streptozotocin (STZ; 2-deoxy-2-(3-(methyl-3-nitrosoureido)-d-glucopyranose) is commonly used as a drug to induce type 1 diabetes in animal models, providing a useful tool for studying the pathology and potential treatment to type 1 diabetes and complications.

STZ is a glucose moiety with a very reactive nitrosourea group that is produced naturally by the mold *Streptomyces* and was first isolated from *Streptomyces achromogenes* fermentation broth. STZ can be synthesized from tetra-O-acetyl glucosamine hydrochloride, D-glucosamine + N-nitrosomethylcarbamyl-azide and from D-glucosamine N-methylurea. STZ possesses broad-spectrum antibacterial, mutagenic and diabetogenic activity and belongs to a family of alkylating antineoplastic drugs called alkylnitrosoureas. This group of compounds was found to be clinically active against a broad range of tumor types including small cell lung cancer, lymphomas, mycosis fungoides, multiple myeloma, glioma and malignant melanoma [5]. However, STZ is not a drug of choice for treatment of cancers due to development of resistance to its genotoxic effects[6]. STZ is highly cytotoxic to the pancreatic beta-cells and therefore is commonly used to induce experimental type 1 diabetes in animal models. There are also many reports using STZ to induce type 2 diabetes. However, the development of hyperglycemia in most of these animal models of type 2 diabetes is primarily a consequence of direct pancreatic beta cell destruction, which is similar to the mechanism of STZ to induce type 1 diabetes, resulting in insulin deficiency rather than insulin resistance [7].

In this book chapter, we will focus on STZ induced type 1 diabetes models. The sensitivity of islet beta cells to STZ is species-specific. Particularly, it has been reported that human islets, in contrast to rat or mouse islets, are much more resistant to the effect of STZ [8]. This was proposed to be due to the different repair and/or defense mechanisms present in islet from different species [9]. Thus different doses and methods are used to induce diabetes in different animal models. Here we will discuss the proper use of STZ to induce type 1 diabetes in different animal models, particularly rodents; the mechanism of action of STZ to result in insulin deficiency and hyperglycemia; and the potential side effect of this drug.

## DOSE AND METHOD OF INDUCING DIABETES USING STZ

Type 1 diabetes can be induced by a single high-dose or multiple low-dose treatment. The merits and pitfalls of these two different methods to induce diabetes are compared in Figure 1. The major merit of single injection is its convenience. This procedure was first introduced in 1963 and has been used in over 7600 PubMed citations, making this the second most used animal model of human disease after the spontaneously hypertensive rat [10]. The amount of STZ used to induce diabetes in the single injection method varies according to the animal species and strains [11]. Generally speaking, dogs are more sensitive to STZ and needs only 30-50 mg/kg to induce diabetes [12-14]. In contrast, mice require higher doses of STZ for inducing diabetes compared with other animals. The dose of STZ is variable among mouse strains with the ICR strain requiring the lowest range (90-150 mg/kg) [15-18], while the C57BL/6 strain needs a higher dose (130-225 mg/kg) [19-22] and the Balb/C strain requires a middle range dose (150 mg/kg) [23]. Due to immunodeficiency [24-26], less STZ (120-140mg/kg) is required by NOD-SCID mice to induce diabetes [24-26]. The dose needed to induce type 1 diabetes in rats can also be strain dependent but is in the general range of 60-85 mg/kg for Sprague-Dowley rats [27-30] and 50-70mg/kg for Wistar rats [31-33]. The single STZ injection, however, causes more side effects and even sudden death in about 10%-20% of the animals due to the rapid elevation of blood glucose and the toxicity of STZ.

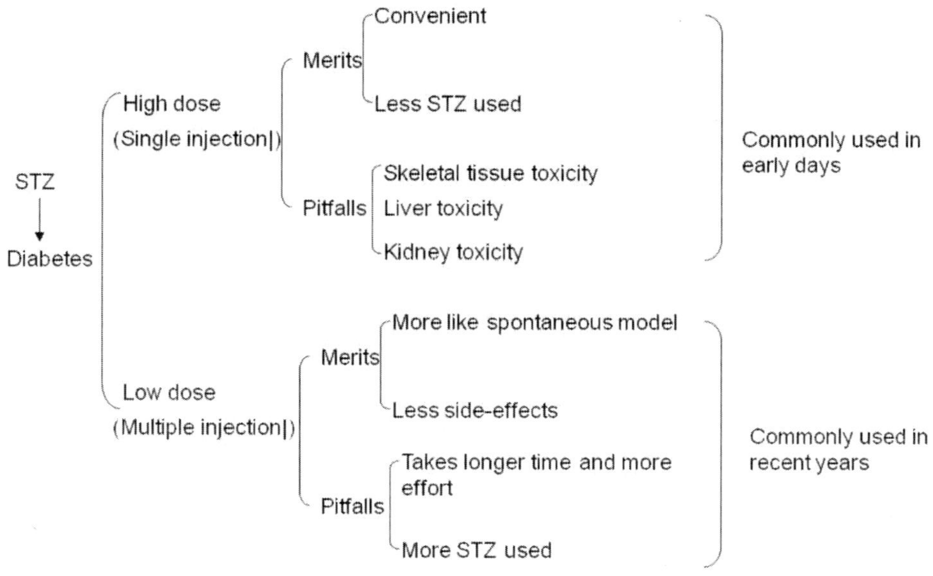


Figure 1. Comparison of the merits and pitfalls of high dose and low dose STZ induced diabetic models.

Given the complications of using single dose STZ, multiple low-dose STZ injection is more commonly used to induce type 1 diabetes, particularly in rodents. The total STZ amount required for multiple low-dose injection is usually higher than the single injection. In most of the mice strains, 5 consecutive daily doses are given totaling approximately 200-300 mg/kg STZ depending on the time and method of injection [34-36]. Typically, mice are given a daily dose of 40 mg/kg to 65 mg/kg STZ to induce type 1 diabetes (as defined by a blood glucose of >300 mg/dl) [11]. This method successfully induces type 1 diabetes in a variety of mouse strains although the resulting degree of hyperglycemia can differ. When injected with 40mg/kg STZ, Balb/c mice had the highest non-fasting blood glucose levels (647 ± 33 mg/dl) when compared to C57BL/6 mice (503 ± 24 mg/dl) and 129/Sv mice (429 ± 28 mg/dl) at 4 weeks after injections. Considering the glucose level in control mice, Balb/c mice are more sensitive to STZ compared to the other two mice strains. Wistar rats can be induced the same way by 40 mg/kg STZ for 5 consecutive days [37]. Type 1 diabetes can be induced in monkeys similarly with a daily injection of STZ (20 mg/kg) for 5 consecutive days, but this is also followed with two additional boosting injections of STZ (25 mg/kg) given 1 week apart[38].

STZ is sometimes used to induce type 2 diabetes either with single high-dose or multiple low-dose treatments. In type 2 diabetes models, the time of dosing is usually different from that of type 1 diabetes, a high dose injection is given on the day of birth, or low-dose STZ injections are combined with a high-fat diet [39]. Other reported experimentally induced type 2 diabetes rodent models using STZ in both routine pharmacological screening and mechanistic diabetes-linked research trials in the past few decades include: adult STZ/alloxan rat models, nicotinamide/STZ models, and the STZ-induced progressive diabetic model etc. However, these methods are not as popular as spontaneously or high fat diet induced type 2 diabetic rodent models.

The method of STZ injection can vary depending upon the study. Intraperitoneal injection is most commonly used to induce diabetes in rodents because it is easier than intravenous injection. Intravenous injection is generally used in larger animals because of their larger veins, somewhat less STZ is required, and higher absorption efficiency is achieved. The dose of STZ for intravenous injection is approximately 90% of that for intraperitoneal injection [11]. While some studies examine the earliest effects of STZ on the pancreas at 6 hours[40], most investigations in rodents examine the complications of diabetes over the course of the condition for 2-6 weeks and sometimes 8 weeks after the first STZ injection. However, there are also some studies that extend this time out to 24 weeks to determine the mechanisms of the chronic complications of diabetes such as neuropathy, retinopathy and nephropathy. In the latter case, insulin injections are sometimes given to extend the survival of the diabetic rodent.

## One Typical Method to Induce Type 1 Diabetes in C57B/6 Mice

One typical method to induced type 1 diabetes in 12 week old C57B/6 mice is listed here. STZ is given at 50mg/kg in 0.1 M citrate buffer by intraperitoneal injection for five consecutive days. Diabetes is confirmed 12 days after the first injection with an AccuChek compact glucometer (Roche, Nutley, NJ) and a drop of blood collected from the saphenous vein. Blood glucose levels over 300 mg/dl are considered diabetic.

STZ degrades rapidly in solution and therefore must be stored below -20°C in a powder form. Typically, STZ is aliquoted in 1.5 ml microtubes with 13 mg in each tube (enough for 10 mice injections) immediately once it is received. This amount is calculated based on that the average of body weight of the mice is 26g. STZ is most stable at pH 4.5 and degrades rapidly in alkaline solutions, forming diazomethane, an alkylating agent [41]. Therefore, for inducing diabetes in mice, STZ is usually dissolved right before injection in filter sterilized 0.1 M citrate buffer (pH 4.5). Citrate buffer should be prepared freshly for each new experiment and keep at 4°C. The recipe of dissolving citrate buffer is as follows.

5.2g citric acid
7.4g sodium citrate
Add 300ml double distilled $H_2O$
pH should be around 4.5.
Add water to 500ml
Sterilize the solution using 0.2 μm filters.

One ml filtered citrate buffer was added to each tube with 13 mg STZ and mixed thoroughly. Inject 100μl of the solution intraperitoneally into each mouse. During the period of mouse injections, keep the needle/syringe on ice in between mouse injections to keep the solution as cold as possible. If the bodyweight of the mouse is different from 26g, adjust the injecting volume accordingly.

## Mechanism of Action of STZ

The selective toxicity of STZ on pancreatic beta cells and its effect on inducing diabetes are related to the similarity between its structure and the structure of glucose moiety, which enables STZ to enter the beta cell through the low affinity GLUT2 glucose transporter in the plasma membrane of pancreatic beta cells [42]. Cells expressing GLUT1 but not GLUT2 transporters are not susceptible to the toxicity of STZ[8]. Because the GLUT2 transporter is not only expressed by pancreatic beta cells but also by other cells such as adipocytes, hepatocytes and renal tubular cells[43], STZ treatment can potentially cause secondary effects including liver and kidney damage of variable degrees depending on the dose of STZ [44]. The different sensitivity of GLUT2 expressing cells results from the different levels of GLUT2 expression [8]. Therefore, using the lowest possible dose of STZ to induce diabetes is very critical in studying the diabetes and complications in an accurate way without causing additional non-diabetic symptoms.

Through decades of diabetes research, the toxicity mechanism and mode of action of STZ was found to be multifaceted. Basically, the cytotoxicity of STZ was proposed to be related to its capacity to affect the insulin secretion function of pancreatic beta cells, particularly by inducing DNA damage and affecting DNA synthesis [45]. However, in the presence of 50 μg of STZ per ml in cultured cells, protein and RNA synthesis are unaffected or inhibited very moderately [41]. STZ induces two distinct forms of cell death in pancreatic beta cells in a concentration dependent manner. At lower doses, STZ can trigger DNA damage and ultimately cause apoptosis of beta cells, whereas at higher doses of STZ, the predominant mode of cell death is necrosis [46]. This was confirmed at cell level using INS-1 cells, a pancreatic beta cell line. The cells were exposed to different concentrations of STZ for variable periods and it was found that higher rates of apoptosis were observed when cells were exposed to low dose (15 mM) STZ for 1 hr followed by 24 hrs recovery period, while higher rates of necrosis were observed with higher doses of STZ (30 mM) [46]. It is notable that at lower doses, beta cells remain viable but stayed in a status of long-term functional defect due to a preferential deficiency of mitochondrial oxidative metabolism [47]. Studying STZ toxicity using HepG2 cells indicated that the toxicity is at least in part, caused by the increase in ROS/RNS production, oxidative stress and mitochondrial dysfunction [48]. These effects inhibit cell mitosis and proliferation at a much lower level and cause cell death at a higher level [49].

*In vivo*, depending on the dose, STZ can impair pancreatic beta cell function and induce diabetes in animals through several different mechanisms. At higher dose, STZ typically targets beta cells by its alkylating property of its methylnitrosourea moiety, especially at the $O^6$ position of guanine, corresponding to that of cytotoxic nitrosouresa compounds [47] [50]. This causes DNA methylation, which leads to the break of DNA trands and impairs the normal physiological function of DNA. In order to repair the damaged DNA, PARP is over-activated and depletes cellular NAD+ and ATP stores [51-53]. This depletion of energy stores is ultimately responsible for beta cell death[54] by necrosis [47]. Thus inhibitors of poly ADP-ribosylation which can prevent the DNA methylation is able to prevent STZ induced beta cell death[55]. This was also confirmed by the observation that mice deficient in PARP are resistant to beta cell death when treated with STZ, though DNA fragmentation exists. Methylation of beta cell proteins was further shown to contribute to the functional defects of beta cells [47]. Another possible mechanism of STZ induced pancreatic beta cell death involves oxidative stress induced by free radicals, NO and reactive oxygen species [56-58]. These were primarily due to the malfunction of mitochondria induced by STZ. A marked increase in mitochondrial oxidative stress in targeted tissue of STZ treated rats was observed [57]. With multiple low doses, STZ causes the release of glutamic acid decarboxylase autoantigens, which may elicit an immune and inflammatory reaction. Under this condition, inflammatory infiltrates including lymphocytes in the pancreatic islet cause the destruction of beta cells and induce the hyperglycemic state [59].

STZ can also inhibit several enzymes, such as O-GlcNAcase, involved in cellular processes[45]. This is another mechanism by which STZ could cause beta cell apoptosis as the inhibition of O-GlcNAcase can lead to intracellular hyper O-GlcNAcylation of proteins which in turn results in the onset of stress response and lead to apoptosis [45, 60]. Though it was found that STZ inhibited DNA synthesis, several enzymes involved in DNA synthesis (such as deoxycytidine kinase, thymidine kinase, DNA polymerase, and thymidylate synthetase) were only moderately inhibited at very high levels of STZ [49].

## Effect of STZ on other Physiological Parameters and Potential Side Effects

STZ induced diabetic models widely used to study the pathology of diabetes and diabetic complications such as osteoporosis, nephropathy, neuropathy and retinopathy. The severity of type 1 diabetes is related to the model used. High dose STZ treatment causes a greater increase in blood glucose levels at early but not late time points compared to low-dose STZ [61]. As STZ can have toxicity effects, it is important to confirm physiologic results obtained from the STZ induced diabetic model with spontaneous models. Using bone pathology as an example, the effects observed in multiple low-dose STZ-induced diabetic mice, marked by a significant decrease in bone volume fraction and decreased levels of markers of osteoblast maturation and increased levels of markers of adipogensis [62, 63], are also observed in spontaneous diabetic model [4]. Consistent results were also achieved in STZ induced young mice and Ins2-akita mice which are a novel spontaneous diabetic mouse model for studying the juvenile diabetes [64]. These studies support the STZ model as being physiologically relevant for the study of type 1 diabetic bone loss. In rats, evidence suggests that administration of STZ to young rats results in impaired skeletal muscle fiber growth independent of the diabetic phenotype. However, these findings were done by single high dose injection of STZ to the rats [65]. Therefore, this conclusion might need further investigation using multiple low-dose STZ to induce diabetes. In addition, increased osteoclastogenesis markers were observed in high-STZ-rodents, which is not commonly observed in spontaneous diabetic models. This may explain some of the disparity between existing studies regarding the role of osteoclasts in diabetic bone pathology.

High-dose STZ can have toxic effect on liver and kidney [66-68], which are the sites of greatest drug accumulation. High-dose STZ can directly cause liver inflammation [61] and subsequent malfunction[67]. Microarray analysis indicated that cycle/apoptosis related genes, immune/allergy related genes and stress response/xenobiotic metabolism related genes in liver cells of the STZ treated mice were upregulated prior to the elevation of the serum glucose levels [69]. This is consistent with the previously reported hepatic changes such as lipid peroxidation, mitochondrial swelling and inhibition of hepatocyte proliferation observed before the development of hyperglycemia [70]. STZ was also shown to have a direct action on neurons and modulate the expression and function of TRPV1 causing hyperalgesia [71]. However, most of these observations of secondary toxicity effects were only seen in high-STZ-dosed rodents. The body parameters of low-dose STZ induced diabetic rodents are similar to the corresponding spontaneous models [4, 61]. When low-dose STZ (45 mg/kg) is used, the majority of functional renal disturbances, changes in renal weight, GFR, urinary albumin excretion and tissue oxygen tension, reflect the diabetic condition rather than the direct side effect of STZ [72].

## Conclusion

Though STZ itself can cause carcinogenesis and renal, hepatic and muscle myoblast toxicity, these side effects can be minimized or completely avoided by using lower doses. It is for this reason that STZ has been wildly used to study the pathology of diabetes and complications. Therefore, the multiple low-dose STZ mouse models serve as useful tools to examine mechanisms of type 1 diabetes and its complications.

## REFERENCES


[1] Sabin, M.A., F.J. Cameron, and G.A. Werther, Type 1 diabetes--still the commonest form of diabetes in children. *Aust Fam Physician,* 2009. *38*(9): p. 695-7.

[2] Urban, A.D. and M. Grey, Type 1 diabetes. *Nurs Clin North Am,* 2006. *41*(4): p. 513-30, vi.

[3] Coe, L.M., J. Zhang, and L.R. McCabe, Both spontaneous Ins2(+/-) and streptozotocin-induced type I diabetes cause bone loss in young mice. J Cell Physiol.

[4] Botolin, S. and L.R. McCabe, Bone loss and increased bone adiposity in spontaneous and pharmacologically induced diabetic mice. *Endocrinology,* 2007. *148*(1): p. 198-205.

[5] Bolzan, A. D. and M.S. Bianchi. Genotoxicity of Streptozotocin. Mutation Research, 2002. 512(2002): p. 121-134.

[6] Capucci, M.S., M.E. Hoffmann, and A.T. Natarajan, Streptozotocin-induced genotoxic effects in Chinese hamster cells: the resistant phenotype of V79 cells. *Mutat Res,* 1995. *347*(2): p. 79-85.

[7] Rerup, C.C., Drugs producing diabetes through damage of the insulin secreting cells. *Pharmacol Rev,* 1970. *22*(4): p. 485-518.

[8] Hosokawa, M., W. Dolci, and B. Thorens, Differential sensitivity of GLUT1- and GLUT2-expressing beta cells to streptozotocin. *Biochem Biophys Res Commun,* 2001. *289*(5): p. 1114-7.

[9] Eizirik, D.L., et al., Major species differences between humans and rodents in the susceptibility to pancreatic beta-cell injury. *Proc Natl Acad Sci U S A,* 1994. *91*(20): p. 9253-6.

[10] Wei, M., et al., The streptozotocin-diabetic rat as a model of the chronic complications of human diabetes. *Heart Lung Circ,* 2003. *12*(1): p. 44-50.

[11] Sakata, N., et al., Animal models of diabetes mellitus for islet transplantation. *Exp Diabetes Res. 2012*: p. 256707.

[12] Alkharfy, K.M., Influence of overt diabetes mellitus on cyclosporine pharmacokinetics in a canine model. *Exp Diabetes Res,* 2009. *2009*: p. 363787.

[13] Matsuo, S., et al., Emphysematous cystitis in a chemically-induced diabetic dog. *J Toxicol Pathol*, 2009. *22*(4): p. 289-92.

[14] Zhu, S., et al., Effects of intrahepatic bone-derived mesenchymal stem cells autotransplantation on the diabetic Beagle dogs. *J Surg Res. 168*(2): p. 213-23.

[15] Tahara, A., et al., Antidiabetic effects of SGLT2-selective inhibitor ipragliflozin in streptozotocin-nicotinamide-induced mildly diabetic mice. *J Pharmacol Sci. 120*(1): p. 36-44.

[16] Kim, H.K., Ecklonia cava Inhibits Glucose Absorption and Stimulates Insulin Secretion in Streptozotocin-Induced Diabetic Mice. *Evid Based Complement Alternat Med. 2012*: p. 439294.

[17] Kim, M.J. and H.K. Kim, Insulinotrophic and hypolipidemic effects of Ecklonia cava in streptozotocin-induced diabetic mice. *Asian Pac J Trop Med.* 5(5): p. 374-9.

[18] Matsuyama-Yokono, A., et al., ASP8497 is a novel selective and competitive dipeptidyl peptidase-IV inhibitor with antihyperglycemic activity. *Biochem Pharmacol,* 2008. *76*(1): p. 98-107.

[19] Yang, B., et al., Bosentan ameliorates the expression of fibrotic related growth factors and collagen-1 in diabetic mice. *Anadolu Kardiyol Derg. 12*(8): p. 621-7.

[20] Zhang, Y., et al., Regeneration of pancreatic non-beta endocrine cells in adult mice following a single diabetes-inducing dose of streptozotocin. *PLoS One. 7*(5): p. e36675.

[21] Wang, C.D., et al., Effect of a novel proteoglycan PTP1B inhibitor from Ganoderma lucidum on the amelioration of hyperglycaemia and dyslipidaemia in db/db mice. *Br J Nutr. 108*(11): p. 2014-25.

[22] Wang, T., et al., Danshensu ameliorates the cognitive decline in streptozotocin-induced diabetic mice by attenuating advanced glycation end product-mediated neuroinflammation. *J Neuroimmunol. 245*(1-2): p. 79-86.

[23] Ulugol, A., et al., 5-HT7 receptor activation attenuates thermal hyperalgesia in streptozocin-induced diabetic mice. *Pharmacol Biochem Behav. 102*(2): p. 344-8.

[24] Banga, A., et al., In vivo reprogramming of Sox9+ cells in the liver to insulin-secreting ducts. *Proc Natl Acad Sci U S A. 109*(38): p. 15336-41.

[25] Bose, B., et al., Human embryonic stem cell differentiation into insulin secreting beta-cells for diabetes. *Cell Biol Int. 36*(11): p. 1013-20.

[26] Han, J., et al., Remission of diabetes by insulin gene therapy using a hepatocyte-specific and glucose-responsive synthetic promoter. *Mol Ther. 19*(3): p. 470-8.

[27] Blaes, N., et al., Bradykinin inhibits high glucose- and growth factor-induced collagen synthesis in mesangial cells through the B2-kinin receptor. *Am J Physiol Renal Physiol. 303*(2): p. F293-303.

[28] Verma, A.K., et al., Flavone-based novel antidiabetic and antidyslipidemic agents. *J Med Chem. 55*(10): p. 4551-67.

[29] Tirgan, N., et al., Nicotine exposure exacerbates development of cataracts in a type 1 diabetic rat model. *Exp Diabetes Res. 2012*: p. 349320.

[30] Talbot, S., et al., Activation of kinin B1 receptor evokes hyperthermia through a vagal sensory mechanism in the rat. *J Neuroinflammation. 9*: p. 214.

[31] Salum, E., et al., Effect of vitamin D on aortic remodeling in streptozotocin-induced diabetes. *Cardiovasc Diabetol. 11*: p. 58.

[32] Peres, G.B., et al., Lysosomal enzymes are decreased in the kidney of diabetic rats. *Biochim Biophys Acta. 1832*(1): p. 85-95.

[33] Khaliq, F., et al., Terminalia arjuna improves cardiovascular autonomic neuropathy in streptozotocin-induced diabetic rats. *Cardiovasc Toxicol. 13*(1): p. 68-76.

[34] Tie, L., et al., Genistein accelerates refractory wound healing by suppressing superoxide and FoxO1/iNOS pathway in type 1 diabetes. *J Nutr Biochem. 24*(1): p. 88-96.

[35] Ochman, A.R., et al., The Lyn kinase activator MLR-1023 is a novel insulin receptor potentiator that elicits a rapid-onset and durable improvement in glucose homeostasis in animal models of type 2 diabetes. *J Pharmacol Exp Ther. 342*(1): p. 23-32.

[36] Li, Y.Y., et al., Adipose-derived mesenchymal stem cells ameliorate STZ-induced pancreas damage in type 1 diabetes. *Biomed Mater Eng. 22*(1-3): p. 97-103.

[37] Arambasic, J., et al., Alpha-lipoic acid upregulates antioxidant enzyme gene expression and enzymatic activity in diabetic rat kidneys through an O-GlcNAc-dependent mechanism. *Eur J Nutr. 52*(5): p. 1461-73.

[38] Wei, L., et al., Induction of diabetes with signs of autoimmunity in primates by the injection of multiple-low-dose streptozotocin. *Biochem Biophys Res Commun. 412*(2): p. 373-8.

[39] Srinivasan, K., et al., Combination of high-fat diet-fed and low-dose streptozotocin-treated rat: a model for type 2 diabetes and pharmacological screening. *Pharmacol Res,* 2005. *52*(4): p. 313-20.

[40] West, E., O.R. Simon, and E.Y. Morrison, Streptozotocin alters pancreatic beta-cell responsiveness to glucose within six hours of injection into rats. *West Indian Med J,* 1996. *45*(2): p. 60-2.

[41] Reusser, F., Mode of action of streptozotocin. *J Bacteriol,* 1971. *105*(2): p. 580-8.

[42] Elsner, M., et al., Relative importance of transport and alkylation for pancreatic beta-cell toxicity of streptozotocin. *Diabetologia,* 2000. *43*(12): p. 1528-33.

[43] Thorens, B., et al., Cloning and functional expression in bacteria of a novel glucose transporter present in liver, intestine, kidney, and beta-pancreatic islet cells. *Cell,* 1988. *55*(2): p. 281-90.

[44] Delaney, C.A., et al., Comparison of inhibition of glucose-stimulated insulin secretion in rat islets of Langerhans by streptozotocin and methyl and ethyl nitrosoureas and methanesulphonates. Lack of correlation with nitric oxide-releasing or O6-alkylating ability. *Biochem Pharmacol,* 1995. *50*(12): p. 2015-20.

[45] He, Y., et al., Structural insight into the mechanism of streptozotocin inhibition of O-GlcNAcase. *Carbohydr Res,* 2009. *344*(5): p. 627-31.

[46] Saini, K.S., et al., Streptozotocin at low doses induces apoptosis and at high doses causes necrosis in a murine pancreatic beta cell line, INS-1. *Biochem Mol Biol Int,* 1996. *39*(6): p. 1229-36.

[47] Lenzen, S., The mechanisms of alloxan- and streptozotocin-induced diabetes. *Diabetologia,* 2008. *51*(2): p. 216-26.

[48] Raza, H. and A. John, Streptozotocin-Induced Cytotoxicity, Oxidative Stress and Mitochondrial Dysfunction in Human Hepatoma HepG2 Cells. *Int J Mol Sci. 13*(5): p. 5751-67.

[49] Bhuyan, B.K., The action of streptozotocin on mammalian cells. *Cancer Res,* 1970. *30*(7): p. 2017-23.

[50] Dufrane, D., et al., Streptozotocin-induced diabetes in large animals (pigs/primates): role of GLUT2 transporter and beta-cell plasticity. *Transplantation,* 2006. *81*(1): p. 36-45.

[51] Uchigata, Y., et al., Protection by superoxide dismutase, catalase, and poly(ADP-ribose) synthetase inhibitors against alloxan- and streptozotocin-induced islet DNA strand breaks and against the inhibition of proinsulin synthesis. *J Biol Chem,* 1982. *257*(11): p. 6084-8.

[52] Yamamoto, H., Y. Uchigata, and H. Okamoto, DNA strand breaks in pancreatic islets by in vivo administration of alloxan or streptozotocin. *Biochem Biophys Res Commun,* 1981. *103*(3): p. 1014-20.

[53] Yamamoto, H., Y. Uchigata, and H. Okamoto, Streptozotocin and alloxan induce DNA strand breaks and poly(ADP-ribose) synthetase in pancreatic islets. *Nature,* 1981. *294*(5838): p. 284-6.

[54] Wilson, G.L., et al., Mechanisms of nitrosourea-induced beta-cell damage. Activation of poly (ADP-ribose) synthetase and cellular distribution. *Diabetes*, 1988. *37*(2): p. 213-6.

[55] Stauffacher, W., et al., Streptozotocin diabetes: time course of irreversible B-cell damage; further observations on prevention by nicotinamide. *Proc Soc Exp Biol Med,* 1970. *133*(1): p. 194-200.

[56] Friederich, M., P. Hansell, and F. Palm, Diabetes, oxidative stress, nitric oxide and mitochondria function. *Curr Diabetes Rev,* 2009. *5*(2): p. 120-44.

[57] Raza, H., et al., Elevated mitochondrial cytochrome P450 2E1 and glutathione S-transferase A4-4 in streptozotocin-induced diabetic rats: tissue-specific variations and roles in oxidative stress. *Diabetes,* 2004. *53*(1): p. 185-94.

[58] Raza, H., et al., Impaired mitochondrial respiratory functions and oxidative stress in streptozotocin-induced diabetic rats. *Int J Mol Sci. 12*(5): p. 3133-47.

[59] Paik, S.G., N. Fleischer, and S.I. Shin, Insulin-dependent diabetes mellitus induced by subdiabetogenic doses of streptozotocin: obligatory role of cell-mediated autoimmune processes. *Proc Natl Acad Sci U S A,* 1980. *77*(10): p. 6129-33.

[60] Konrad, R.J., et al., The potential mechanism of the diabetogenic action of streptozotocin: inhibition of pancreatic beta-cell O-GlcNAc-selective N-acetyl-beta-D-glucosaminidase. *Biochem J*, 2001. *356*(Pt 1): p. 31-41.

[61] Motyl, K. and L.R. McCabe, Streptozotocin, type I diabetes severity and bone. *Biol Proced Online,* 2009. *11*: p. 296-315.

[62] Martin, L.M. and L.R. McCabe, Type I diabetic bone phenotype is location but not gender dependent. *Histochem Cell Biol,* 2007. *128*(2): p. 125-33.

[63] Botolin, S., et al., Increased bone adiposity and peroxisomal proliferator-activated receptor-gamma2 expression in type I diabetic mice. *Endocrinology,* 2005. *146*(8): p. 3622-31.

[64] Coe, L.M., J. Zhang, and L.R. McCabe, Both spontaneous Ins2(+/-) and streptozotocin-induced type I diabetes cause bone loss in young mice. *J Cell Physiol. 228*(4): p. 689-95.

[65] Johnston, A.P., et al., Streptozotocin induces G2 arrest in skeletal muscle myoblasts and impairs muscle growth in vivo. *Am J Physiol Cell Physiol,* 2007. *292*(3): p. C1033-40.

[66] Weiss, R.B., Streptozocin: a review of its pharmacology, efficacy, and toxicity. *Cancer Treat Rep,* 1982. *66*(3): p. 427-38.

[67] Schein, P.S. and S. Loftus, Streptozotocin: depression of mouse liver pyridine nucleotides. *Cancer Res,* 1968. *28*(8): p. 1501-6.

[68] Graham, M.L., et al., Refining the high-dose streptozotocin-induced diabetic non-human primate model: an evaluation of risk factors and outcomes. *Exp Biol Med (Maywood). 236*(10): p. 1218-30.

[69] Kume, E., et al., Gene expression profiling in streptozotocin treated mouse liver using DNA microarray. *Exp Toxicol Pathol,* 2005. *56*(4-5): p. 235-44.

[70] Kume, E., et al., Hepatic changes in the acute phase of streptozotocin (SZ)-induced diabetes in mice. *Exp Toxicol Pathol,* 2004. *55*(6): p. 467-80.

[71] Pabbidi, R.M., et al., Direct role of streptozotocin in inducing thermal hyperalgesia by enhanced expression of transient receptor potential vanilloid 1 in sensory neurons. *Mol Pharmacol,* 2008. *73*(3): p. 995-1004.

[72] Palm, F., et al., Differentiating between effects of streptozotocin per se and subsequent hyperglycemia on renal function and metabolism in the streptozotocin-diabetic rat model. *Diabetes Metab Res Rev,* 2004. *20*(6): p. 452-9.

In: Streptozotocin: Uses, Mechanism of Action and Side Effects ISBN: 978-1-63117-255-7
Editor: Elizabeth L. Gauthier 

*Chapter 3*

# Cognitive Impairment Induced by Streptozotocin: An Experimental Link between Diabetes and Alzheimer's Disease

***Patrícia Nardin[1], Ana Carolina Tramontina[2], Patrícia Sesterheim[3], Leticia Rodrigues[1], Regina Biasibetti[1] and Carlos-Alberto Gonçalves[1,*]***

[1]Biochemistry Department of Federal University of Rio Grande do Sul (UFRGS), Porto Alegre, Brazil

[2]State University of Rio Grande do Sul (UERGS)

[3]State Foundation of Research and Production for Health (FEPPS-RS)

## Abstract

Diabetes mellitus is a common and growing metabolic disorder that is associated with chronic complications, particularly affecting kidney, vessels and neural tissues. Cell targets in the central nervous system include neurons and astrocytes. Brain commitment has been confirmed by cognitive impairment in the diabetic population and experimental models of diabetes.

In addition, we know that the risk for Alzheimer´s disease is increased in diabetic individuals. Glucosamine-nitrosourea streptozotocin (STZ) administration has been widely used to induce experimental diabetes, due to its toxicity to β-cells of the islets of Langerhans.

This compound does not cross the blood brain barrier, but the brain damage associated with ensuing diabetes can, therefore, be studied. Conversely, intracerebroventricular injection of STZ has been used as a model of dementia, where many characteristics of Alzheimer´s disease are observed to include β-amyloid deposits. In this chapter, we will discuss the link between the cognitive impairment in diabetes mellitus and Alzheimer´s disease, using the experimental evidence obtained using STZ administration and focusing on the alterations in astrocytes, the most abundant glial cells that are intimately connected (both structurally and metabolically) to neurons.

* Corresponding author: casg@ufrgs.br.

# 1. Introduction

Although we have improved the management of diabetes mellitus (DM), the mortality due to cardiovascular and renal complications is still very high [1] and elderly diabetic individuals demonstrate cognitive impairment and an elevated risk of dementia [2–4]. Evidence from epidemiological and experimental studies suggest a close association between DM and cognitive deficit, which is frequently associated with Alzheimer's disease (AD).

Experimental cognitive impairment, induced by streptozotocin (STZ), has been observed during the last 20 years [5]. STZ, or 2-deoxy-2-(3-(methyl-3-nitrosoureido))-D-glucopyranose, is used therapeutically to kill neuroendocrine tumor cells (e.g. islet cell carcinoma) [6] and, experimentally, to induce DM and also Alzheimer's type dementia [7]. While type-1 DM is usually induced in rodents by a single large intraperitoneal dose of STZ, type-2 DM requires administration of a small dose of STZ and additional procedures, such as fructose- or fat-enriched diets [8]. Although the toxic mechanism of STZ is not fully understood, we know that it depends on transport by GLUT-2 [9] and involves methylation of DNA and nitrosative stress [10].

Herein, we will broach the effect and mechanism of STZ in both types of DM and Alzheimer´s type dementia, although evidence suggests a particular association between type 2 DM and AD. In this chapter, we will discuss the link between the cognitive impairment in diabetes mellitus and Alzheimer´s disease, using the experimental evidence obtained with STZ administration and focusing on the alterations in astrocytes, the most abundant glial cells that are intimately connected (both structurally and metabolically) to neurons.

# 2. Cognitive Impairment in Diabetes Mellitus

Although cognitive impairment and alteration of glucose metabolism are associated with age, the causal link between them is debatable. At least three biochemical alterations have been studied and associated with cognitive deficit in DM: vascular alterations, particularly atherosclerosis (reducing molecular traffic to and from the brain), insulin resistance and poor glucose regulation. In some studies, cognitive impairment was observed even after the control of vascular alterations [11]. Moreover, young diabetic individuals (type 1 DM) demonstrate cognitive deficits prior to the occurrence of clear vascular alterations and independently of episodes of hypoglycemia [12]. However, microvascular alterations are currently pathological elements observed in Alzheimer´s disease and vascular dementia [4].

STZ-induced DM presents alterations in vascular response to neurotransmitters in the retina [13] and mesenteric microvessels [14]. It is important mention that the STZ administration in the latter study was performed in neonate rats, as a model of type 2 DM. These data suggest that brain vascular alterations, induced by STZ, could support cognitive deficits observed in DM. Moreover, it is important to emphasize that altered vascular permeability is intimately related to other possible biochemical alterations responsible for cognitive impairment: insulin resistance and poor glucose regulation (see Figure 1).

In STZ-induced DM, spatial learning impairments have been observed for tasks dependent on hippocampal integrity [15]. In support of these data, biochemical and electrophysiological alterations have been described in these rats [16, 17]. Moreover, specific astroglial changes were observed in GFAP [18, 19] and gap junctional communication [20]. In high-fat fed rats, STZ was able to induce a type 2 DM, characterized by hyperglycemia, hyperlipidemia and insulin resistance. These animals exhibited cognitive impairment and changes in hippocampal cell signaling [21]. Assuming that STZ does not cross the blood brain barrier in the DM model, it may be suggested that the resulting insulin resistance and/or hyperglycemia underlie the alterations in the neurons and glial cells. In fact, insulin signaling in neurons and glial cells modulates many activities including survival, proliferation and synaptic plasticity [22, 23] and, therefore, STZ could affect brain without coming into contact with it. Moreover, the high glucose levels induced by STZ, directly or indirectly, for example via methylglyoxal [24] or advanced glycation end products [25] are able to affect cell signaling.

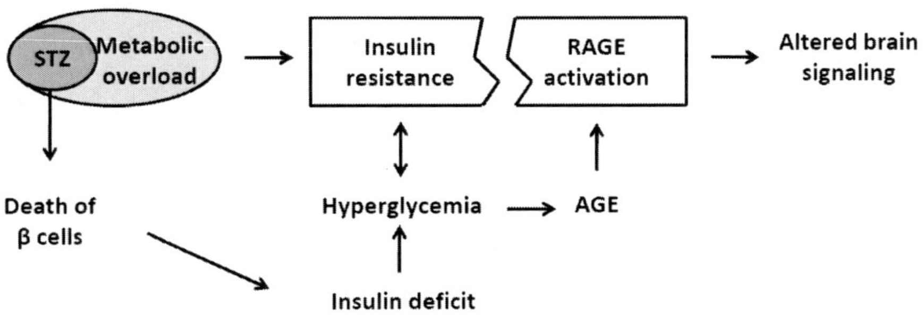


Figure 1. *Putative links between STZ, diabetes mellitus and cognitive impairment.* STZ directly destroys beta cells of Langerhans islets leading to type 1 DM. STZ also is able to cause type 2 diabetes, when associated with metabolic overload (e.g. high fat diet). The resulting hyperglycemia and advanced glycation end products (AGE), in turn, result in decrease of insulin mediated communication (insulin resistance) and activation of RAGE, respectively. Both pathways are involved in altered cell signaling in brain tissue and cognitive impairment.

In summary, STZ induces a direct and permanent decrease in insulin mimicking type 1 DM. In addition, during the neonatal phase or when given together with a high-sucrose or high-fat diet, STZ induces a partial destruction of beta cells, which leads to a compensatory hyperinsulinemia and further insulin resistance. Both types of DM result in a lack of cell signaling mediated by insulin.

This results in high glucose levels, through mediated by products such as advanced glycation end products (AGE) active receptors for AGE (RAGE). RAGE activation mediates the inflammatory process observed in vessels and kidneys in DM [26]. In the brain and peripheral nerves, both alterations in cell signaling (decrease in insulin signaling and increase in RAGE signaling) could be involved in the cognitive impairment observed in DM and STZ-induced DM (see Figure 1).

## 3. Neurochemical Alterations Induced by STZ-Diabetes Mellitus

The STZ-diabetes animal model, regardless of type, is associated with various brain alterations. It has already been emphasized that the type and the extent of the modifications are a function of both, severity and duration of the diabetes [27]. Neuronal and glial abnormalities in several brain areas have been observed during STZ-induced diabetes [28]. Astrocytes play critical roles in central nervous system (CNS) homeostasis, including regulation of neuronal and synaptic activities, maintenance of the blood-brain barrier, energy supply, protection against oxidative damage, production of growth factors as well as the control of ion and neurotransmitter concentration, among many others [29, 30].

In response to any kind of injury to CNS, astrocytes change their appearance. This phenomenon is known as reactive gliosis or astrogliosis. A key indicator commonly used as a marker of glial reactivity is the glial fibrillary acidic protein (GFAP), an astrocyte intermediate filament protein [31]. On the hand, many studies have shown an increase in the number of GFAP+ astrocytes [32, 33] and in the GFAP levels in various brain regions (hippocampus, cortex and/or cerebellum) [32, 34–36]. However, no differences were seen in the number of astrocytes and a significant decrease in GFAP levels was demonstrated in STZ-diabetic rats [37, 38] following insulin treatment [18].

Oxidative stress, an imbalance between intracellular levels of oxidants and antioxidants, is observed in DM [39]. Hyperglycemia may cause oxidative stress, producing reactive oxygen species that react with cellular components and contribute to increased neuronal death through protein oxidation, DNA damage and peroxidation of membrane lipids [40]. Studies indicate that there exists a presence of oxidative damage and decrease in the antioxidant system in the brain of STZ-induced diabetic rats [20, 41–45].

Hyperglycemia induced in STZ-rodents also enhances the formation of advanced glycation end products (AGEs), the final products of non-enzymatic glycation and oxidation of proteins and lipids [33, 46], as well as the expression of their receptor, RAGE, a member of immunoglobulin superfamily [33, 47, 48]. In addition, the interaction of AGEs with their receptors elicits the production of reactive oxygen species [49].

The insulin receptors (IR) have been demonstrated to be widely distributed in the rat brain [50]. Insulin binding to the brains of STZ-induced diabetic rats was similar to control animal insulin binding and failed to indicate up-regulation of these receptors, when evaluated by means of steady-state binding studies with radiolabeled insulin [51, 52]. However, radioimmunoassay studies have demonstrated that the IR content in the brain of STZ-diabetic rats is increased [53].

The mRNA of IR in the brain of the STZ-induced diabetic rats demonstrated a specific distribution. There were significant differences in the IR mRNA from cortex [54, 55], hypothalamus, amygdale [54] and cerebellum [56] and, although no significant changes in IR gene expression were detected in the hippocampus, the amount of IR protein in this region was reduced [54].

Glutamate is the major excitatory neurotransmitter in the mammalian CNS. In order to maintain the brain homeostasis, glutamate must be removed rapidly from the synaptic cleft by astrocytes. STZ-induced diabetes resulted in a significant increase in glutamate uptake in the glial plasmalemmal vesicle of total brain, and insulin treatment prevented this increase in diabetic animals [18].

However, no significant differences were noted for the GLT-1 or GLAST glutamate transporters in the hippocampus, cortex or cerebellum [37]. The increased glutamate uptake may result from an increased affinity of the transporters for glutamate [57]. Glutamate exerts its effects by interacting with glutamate receptors located in neuronal and glial cells. The glutamate receptors have been divided into two classes: metabotropic (mGluRs 1-8) and ionotropic (NMDA, AMPA and kainate) [58]. The extracellular accumulation of glutamate results in neuronal death by overexcitation of glutamate receptors [59]. Some studies have shown a significant increase in the glutamate content and in the number of glutamate receptors in DM [60, 61]. Additionally, the gene expression of the subunits NMDA 2B, NMDA R1, GluR4-containing AMPA, and mGluR5 receptor was significantly increased in the cerebral cortex of the STZ-diabetic rats [60, 61].

The CNS transmitters play an important role in the regulation of glucose homeostasis [62]. Although the exact means by which neuronal dysfunction occurs subsequent to hypo and hyperglycemia remains unknown, previous reports suggest that variation in the functional regulation of neurotransmitter receptors is associated with cognitive and memory deficits and can lead to neuronal death [63]. Studies have demonstrated that the mRNA levels of muscarinic and nicotinic cholinergic receptors in the cerebral cortex, cerebellum and hippocampus are substantially altered in the STZ-induced diabetic rats, compared to control [55, 56, 64].

Furthermore, GABA receptors (GABA Aα1 and GABA B) gene expression was significantly downregulated [64, 65], while D1 and D2 dopaminergic receptor gene expression was enhanced in the hippocampus of STZ-induced diabetic rats [66].

$Na^+$/ $K^+$ -ATPase is a transmembrane enzyme that is primary responsible for the active transport of sodium and potassium in mammalian cells. This protein is greatly expressed by neurons, consuming 30-60% of brain ATP store and maintains the electrical potential necessary for the excitability of this tissue [67]. STZ causes a significant decrease in the activity $Na^+$/ $K^+$ -ATPase in the various regions of the diabetic rat brain [44, 68–71]. Diabetes induces dysfunction of ion channel activity in nerve terminals [72, 73], where voltage-dependent sodium and potassium currents can influence the excitability of neurons. A decrease in sodium currents and an increase in potassium currents in diabetic neurons was observed in hippocampal slices of STZ-induced diabetic rats, possibly resulting in alterations in learning and memory processing [74].

## 4. The S100B Protein in Diabetes Mellitus

Similarly to GFAP, another protein, S100B, has been used as marker of astroglial activation during brain injury [75]. S100B is a member of a large family of $Ca^{2+}$ - binding proteins of the EF-hand type (helix-loop-helix) (see [76] for a review). Initially, the S100B protein was thought to be specific to the brain, but was later found in many non-neural tissues. In the nervous system, S100B is predominantly expressed and secreted by astrocytes. However, this protein is also expressed in other glial cells, such as olygodendrocytes, Schwann cells, ependymal cells, enteric glial cells and also in certain neuronal populations. Moreover, S100B has been found in various cells of non-neuron tissues including adipocytes, chondrocytes, melanocytes, Langerhans cells, dendritic cells, lymphocyte subpopulations, Leydig cells and skeletal muscle satellite cells [77]. Intracellularly, S100B interacts with different target proteins performing a variety of biological roles, including cytoskeleton regulation, cell proliferation, survival and differentiation [77]. Extracellularly, S100B exerts autocrine or paracrine effects on astrocytes, neurons and microglia [77]. The extracellular role of S100B is mediated by RAGE (receptor for AGEs), a member of the immunoglobulin superfamily [76, 78, 79]. This protein has a trophic or toxic *in vitro* effect, depending on the extracellular concentration of S100B [80].

**Table 1. Changes in the S100B protein in brain tissue of STZ-induced diabetes and STZ-induced dementia rats**

| | *Brain region* | *Time after STZ (in weeks)* | *Change (Method)* | *Reference* |
|---|---|---|---|---|
| **Diabetes** | | | | |
| | Whole [a] | 4-6 | ↑ (WB) | [92] |
| | Hippocampus, cerebral cortex and cerebellum | 6 | ↑ (WB) | [34] |
| | Hippocampus, cerebellum and corpus callosum | 4 and 8 | No change | [37] |
| | Hippocampus, cerebral cortex and cerebellum | 6 | ↑ (WB) | [173] |
| | Olphactory bulb | 8 | No change (IH) | [174] |
| | Hippocampus | 1 and 3 | No change [c] (IH) | [175] |
| | Hippocampus | 6 | No change (WB) | [176] |
| | Hippocampus | 9 | No change (ELISA) | [38] |
| **Dementia** | | | | |
| | Hippocampus | 7 | ↑ (ELISA) | [177] |
| | Hippocampus [b] | 4 | ↑ (LIA) | [178] |
| | Hippocampus | 4 | ↑ (ELISA) | [133] |

Measurements were performed in adult Wistar rats and exceptions are indicated: [a], Sprague Dawlay rats; [b], CF1 mice; [c]A transitory increase as observed in 3 days after STZ administration. WB, Western blotting; IH, immunohistochemistry; LIA, luminescent immune assay; ↑, increase; ↓, decrease.

The S100B level in biological fluids (cerebrospinal fluid-CSF, serum, urine, saliva) has been considered as a biomarker of many pathological conditions [81]. As such, the S100B protein is widely used as a parameter of glial alterations (activation and/or death) in several brain injury conditions, such as trauma [82], ischemia [83], psychiatric disorders [84, 85] and neurodegenerative diseases [86]. However, caution is necessary when considering serum S100B as a glial marker, due to the presence of other extra-brain sources, such as adipocytes, for example, which may contribute to the peripheral levels of this protein [75, 87]. In diabetic patients, serum S100B is decreased in type 2 diabetic patients compared with healthy subjects and type 1 diabetic patients, without significant correlation between serum levels of S100B and the duration of diabetes [88]. In a more recent study, serum S100B was not altered in type 2 DM patients [89], moreover S100B should be considered as a marker as well as a mediator of inflammatory response in DM. In fact, S100B (via RAGE) was reported to be capable of increasing cyclooxygenase -2 expression in human Langerhans islets [90] and NF-kappaB activation in vascular smooth muscle cells [91].

Many authors have reported glial abnormalities in type 1 STZ-induced diabetes in rats, but there are conflicting data regarding the S100B protein, particularly in the hippocampus, a brain region involved in cognitive tasks such as spatial learning and object recognition. S100B mRNA levels were found decreased, while the content of S100B protein was increased in the brain tissue of a type 1 DM model induced by STZ [92]. Most authors found no change in hippocampal S100B (see Table 1), in spite of other glial abnormalities. An increase of S100B has been reported in retinal glial cells and a decrease in enteric glial in the cells of STZ-induced diabetic Sprague-Dawley rats has been described. Only one study reported an increase in CSF S100B in diabetic rats [38]. Assuming that part of the effect of STZ is mediated by hyperglycemia, it is important consider results in neural cells. In a human Müller glial cell line exposed to high glucose (25 mM), both S100B gene expression and the S100B protein content was found to be increased [48]. On the other hand, the S100B content and secretion was found decreased in rat primary cortical astrocytes cultured in high glucose medium (12 mM) [93].

## 5. Alzheimer's Disease, Glucose and Insulin

Alzheimer's disease (AD) is the most common type of dementia, and affects more than 30 million people worldwide [94]. Patients with AD present progressive changes in memory and cognition, as well as behavioral changes [95]. AD is characterized by extensive neuronal loss and gliosis, in addition to two classic lesions: the accumulation of the peptide β-amyloid (βA) and hyperphosphorylation of the tau protein, forming neurofibrillary tangles [96]. Numerous other alterations occur in the AD brain, including cholinergic deficit, alterations in glutamate metabolism, oxidative stress, neuroinflammation [95–97]; however, recently, many research groups have paid more attention to alterations in glucose metabolism and insulin signaling in the brain of AD patients.

AD has been described as an "Insulin-Resistant Brain State" [98], and also as "Type 3 Diabetes" [99]. Cerebral glucose metabolism is markedly altered in AD patients. The expression of GLUT-1 and 3 in the brain of AD patients are reduced [100], which leads to a reduction in glucose uptake, and can produce glucose hypometabolism in the brain. In addition, key glycolytic enzymes demonstrate reduced activities in the AD brain [101, 102]. As a consequence of the reduction in brain glucose metabolism, ATP production in the brain of AD patients can be reduced by around 50%, which compromises many processes that are crucial for cell metabolism [103]. Evidence suggests that insulin plays a key role in the development of glucose hypometabolism in the brain of AD patients. Frölich and collaborators found reduced insulin levels, accompanied by an increase in insulin receptors (IR) expression in the AD brain [104]. Posterior studies demonstrated other major alterations in post-mortem AD brain, such as reduced insulin mRNA [105, 106], reduced IRS-1 and 2 levels and PI3-K and ERK1/2 activities [107]. It should be remembered that insulin signaling plays a key role in tau phosphorylation and βA production, and this finding suggests that alterations in insulin signaling maybe involved in the pathogenesis of AD [98].

# 6. STZ-Induced Dementia

As previously mentioned, STZ is capable of destroying pancreatic beta cells in the periphery, inducing diabetes, but this compound does not cross blood-brain barrier (see Figure 2). However, in subdiabetogenic doses (1-3 mg/kg), and when injected via intracerebroventricular (ICV), this drug generates alterations in the CNS that are very similar to those found in sporadic Alzheimer's Disease (sAD) [17, 108]. To our knowledge, the first report of ICV injection of STZ was in 1989 [109], and since then, many studies have been performed to evaluate the effect of this drug in the CNS. In earlier reports, only the reduction in central glucose metabolism was described [5, 110]; however it is known that many major changes in the CNS occur; as such the ICV-STZ infusion model is a widely-accepted model for sAD [7, 111–113]. After ICV-STZ infusion, severe abnormalities in glucose metabolism develop in the brain. Many research groups have demonstrated a reduction in glucose utilization in different brain areas [114–116]. ICV-STZ causes a reduction in the glucose transporters, GLUT-1 and 3, as well as in glycolytic enzymes activities in the cortex and hippocampus, which leads to an energetic decline in CNS [7, 116, 117].

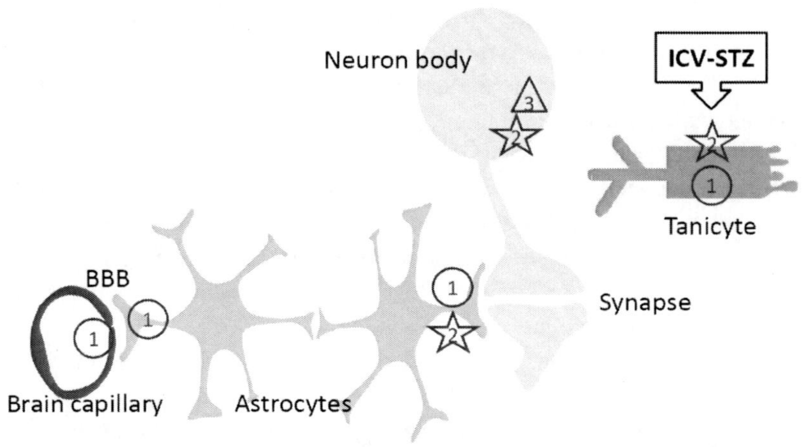


Figure 2. *Schematic representation of the distribution of glucose transporters (GLUT) in brain tissue.* STZ is transported by GLUT-2 and therefore does not cross blood-brain-barrier (BBB). GLUT-2 is observed in glucose sensing neurons (e.g. in hypothalamus), tanycytes (in the wall of brain ventricles and central canal of spinal cord) and perisynaptic astrocytes. Therefore, apparently, intracerebroventricular STZ reaches brain tissue through the tanycytes. Glucose transporters 1, 2 and 3 are represented by circles, stars and triangles, respectively.

In the brain, insulin signaling plays important roles in development and plasticity, affecting learning and memory [118]. It has been suggested that alterations in CNS insulin signaling could be crucial for the development of AD [119–121], and that STZ-induced dementia model is capable of reproducing some of these alterations. ICV-STZ promotes a decrease in insulin receptor expression, an alteration associated with impairment in learning and memory [122]. The downstream steps of insulin signaling are also altered by STZ. It is well established that the PI3K route of insulin signaling is involved in neuronal survival and synaptic plasticity [22]. PI3K is altered by ICV-STZ administration [123]. According to this result, GSK3β overactivation has also been described [123, 124]. GSK3β is the most important kinase involved in tau phosphorylation [125], and its activation leads to an increase in phospho-tau levels, which have been found in the brain of AD patients, and in the brain of STZ-treated animals [123, 126, 127].

As such, STZ administration is very useful for inducing similar biochemical alterations to those observed in sAD, and also to accelerate and exacerbate signals in the transgenic model of AD [128, 129]. STZ models have helped us to understand aspects and evaluate therapeutic strategies for DM and AD. In fact, based on the signaling alterations involved, many therapeutic strategies have been used for STZ-treated animals, including antioxidant and anti-inflammatory compounds (see [130] for a review).

## 7. Neurochemical Alterations in STZ-Induced Dementia

Beyond the metabolic alterations observed in the STZ-dementia model, many neurochemical alterations develop in the CNS. In fact, some of these alterations are a consequence of impaired brain energy metabolism, such as disturbances in cholinergic transmission, which are implicated in the reduction in cognitive capacities. The reduction in glucose metabolism leads to minor acetyl CoA generation, which directly influences the production of choline acetyltransferase (ChAT). In fact, in the STZ-dementia model, there is a marked reduction in ChAT activity in the hippocampus [110, 131, 132]. Furthermore, increased acetylcolinesterase (AChE) has been reported in the ICV-STZ treated brain [124, 131, 133, 134], which contributes to increase the cholinergic deficit in the STZ-dementia model. Together with the cholinergic deficit described, patients with AD present alterations in glutamatergic transmission, with receptor overactivation, reduced levels of glutamate uptake [135], and lower levels of glutamine synthetase (GS) [136]. The STZ-dementia model was able to reproduce the alterations in cholinergic transmission; however, the changes in glutamate were not prominent. Our group found a reduced GS activity in STZ-induced dementia [113, 133]; however the glutamate uptake remains unchanged in the hippocampus of ICV-STZ treated animals [111, 113].

The amyloid deposits that are found in the brains of AD patients are also observed in the STZ-dementia model, but in blood vessels. Salkovic-Petrisic and collaborators related finding amyloid deposits (by congo-red staining) in brain blood vessels at 3 months after STZ administration; however, they did not find typical amyloid plaques [17]. Amyloid deposits were also found on the meningeal wall at 6 and 9 months after STZ administration. Reports have also been made of observations of hyperphosphorylated tau protein in the hippocampus of rats submitted to the STZ-dementia model, at three months after ICV-STZ administration [122].

Astrocytes, the most abundant glial cells in CNS, undergo extensive remodeling in AD [137]. These cells have three specific marker proteins, GFAP, GS, and S100B, and all of these are altered in AD patients. Activated astrocytes, which are characterized by hypertrophy and augmented levels of GFAP and S100B, are found in association with amyloid plaques [138, 139]. However, alterations in S100B expressing cells have been observed even before amyloid deposits in transgenic models of AD [140, 141]. For this reason, S100B has been investigated in AD and other neurodegenerative diseases [75, 85, 142]. An increment of hippocampal S100B content has been related in STZ-induced dementia (see Table 1), but inversely, a decrease in S100B content in cerebrospinal fluid [111, 133] and serum has been seen [143]. It is important to mention that this decrease in CSF S100B in STZ-induced dementia has also been observed in other experimental models using chronic cerebral hypoperfusion and intrahippocampal administration of okadaic acid [144, 145]. Decreased serum S100B has been reported in AD patients [86].

In addition to astroglial damage, STZ also causes damage to neurons and oligodendrocytes. STZ injection causes brain atrophy, as a result of neuron and oligodendrocyte apoptosis [105]. STZ is also capable of causing loss of white matter and damage to myelin in the fornix, at 40 days after injection [146]. Synaptic markers are affected differently, while synaptophysin suffers a marked decrease in the hippocampus at three weeks after ICV-STZ administration, no change has been observed in post-synaptic density 95 (PSD95) [147].

## 8. Changes in Glucose Metabolism Precede Alzheimer's Disease

Brain tissue is highly dependent on glucose and, over the last 20 years, a tight association between glucose consumption and synaptic activity has been established [148]. However, the specific demand for glucose is not limited to the energetic aspect, which in part, might supplied by ketone bodies [149]. Glucose is a substrate for neurotransmitters (glutamate, GABA, acetylcholine), lipids (e.g. all brain cholesterol is synthetized by itself) [150], synthesis and recycling of glutathione - the main antioxidant molecule in brain [151]. Therefore, the altered glucose metabolism in the nervous system could reflect deep alterations in brain energetic, neurotransmission, structure and antioxidant defenses.

It is important to emphasize that all these destinations of glucose in the brain, as well as glucose uptake, are dependent on specific astrocyte pathways. Synthesis of glutamine (for neuronal synthesis of glutamate) is catalyzed by glutamine synthetase, an exclusive astrocyte enzyme in brain [152]. Another specific astrocyte enzyme in the brain is pyruvate carboxylase, which is important for de novo synthesis of glutamate [153]. Cholesterol is exported from astrocytes to neurons by specific lipoproteins containing ApoE [150]. All these aspects of close metabolic interaction between neurons and astrocytes reinforce the importance of understanding the changes in astrocytes markers (e.g. S100B protein) in brain disorders, beyond changes in neuronal markers (e.g. NSE or phospho-tau in Alzheimer´s disease).

Alterations in brain glucose metabolism are a common aspect of Alzheimer's disease (AD)[104] and diabetes mellitus and, in fact, Alzheimer's disease has been proposed by la Monte's group as type 3 DM [121]. This might be explained by the fact that β-amyloid peptide is able to induce neuronal insulin resistance [154]. However, epidemiological studies have revealed cognitive deficits in the elderly diabetic population and that the risk of developing AD is 2-4 times higher in the diabetic population [155, 156]. Growing evidence suggests that glucose metabolism alterations precede the β-amyloid event in AD (see [98, 157]). In agreement, ICV-STZ precedes and eventually leads to increased β-amyloid peptide and tau phosphorylation [130].

At least two alterations have been observed in AD patients in glucose metabolism; decrease in transport and metabolic intracellular dysfunction (particularly mitochondrial) [158]. Using $^{18}$F-fluorodeoxyglucose (FDG) as a tracer in positron emission tomography (PET), regional glucose metabolism was characterized in the hippocampus and other cortical areas [159, 160]. A decrease in glucose uptake was observed in STZ-induced diabetic rats [161]. This impairment in glucose metabolism was also observed in STZ-induced dementia,evaluated by PET/FDG, in non-human primates [162] and in *ex vivo* hippocampal slices of rats evaluated using [2,3-$^{3}$H]deoxy-D-glucose [133].

Oxidative and nitrosative stress, caused by reducing the activity of complexes III, IV and V of the respiratory chain could contribute to brain mitochondrial dysfunction in STZ-induced diabetes mellitus in rats [42], where hippocampal tissue is apparently more affected [163]. Signs of oxidative stress, including decreased glutathione levels and brain mitochondrial dysfunction, have been extensively reported in STZ-induced dementia [39, 44, 51, 108, 112, 131, 164, 165, 166]. However, at this moment, there are no data available to indicate whether neuronal and astrocyte mitochondria exhibit different sensitivities to STZ.

The mechanisms driving the effects of STZ in the diabetes model (by intra peritoneal administration of this compound) and in the dementia model (by intracerebroventricular administration) are unclear. Assuming that STZ entry depends on GLUT-2, a specific population is affected initially, for example beta cells in Langerhans islets in diabetes and some neurons in the dementia model. GLUT-2 has a high $K_M$ when compared to other glucose transporters (GLUT-1, -3 and -4) and is found in peripheral cell types exposed to increased glucose flow, such as enterocytes, tubular cells in the kidneys and hepatocytes [167] and in glucose-sensing cells, such as pancreatic beta cells [168].

In the rat brain, GLUT-2 appears to be widely expressed in many regions, but at low levels [169]. The presence of GLUT-2 with glucokinase in the third ventricle wall and adjacent arcuate nucleus, median eminence, and supraoptic nucleus suggests a role of glucose sensing by these neurons, possibly regulating food behavior [170] (see Figure 2). Moreover, tanicytes [171] and, apparently, perisynaptic astrocytes express this transporter [172]. The involvement of GLUT-2 in Alzheimer´s disease has been supported by experiments employing ICV infusion of 5-thio-d-glucose, an inhibitor of GLUT-2, which causes similar alterations to those observed with STZ [17]. Therefore, it is possible that STZ initially impairs some neurons, astrocytes and tanicytes, and subsequently affects brain cells, possibly also due to insulin resistance and/or RAGE activation.

## CONCLUSION

1. STZ administration leads to insulin resistance and RAGE activation in diabetes mellitus and dementia models.
2. Cognitive impairment is observed in both models and is associated with insulin resistance and RAGE activation.
3. In STZ-induced dementia, insulin resistance precedes beta-amyloid disorder, as occurs in AD.

4. The STZ model of dementia is appropriate for the study of sporadic AD, as it shares several biochemical alterations with the disease, including increased beta-amyloid production and tau phosphorylation.
5. Moreover, STZ administration has been used to accelerate and exacerbate signals in a transgenic model of AD.
6. Glial abnormalities occur in addition to the neuronal alterations induced by STZ, contributing to the cognitive impairment observed.
7. The STZ-model of dementia results in an increase in the S100B protein in the hippocampus, but a decrease in the cerebrospinal fluid.
8. S100B should be considered as a marker of brain injury as well as a mediator of the inflammatory/neurotrophic response (via RAGE) both in diabetes mellitus and in dementia.
9. STZ models have helped in the understanding of aspects DM and AD and to evaluate therapeutic strategies for their treatment.

## References

[1] Van Dieren S, Nöthlings U, van der Schouw YT, et al. (2011) Non-fasting lipids and risk of cardiovascular disease in patients with diabetes mellitus. *Diabetologia* 54:73–77. doi: 10.1007/s00125-010-1945-z.

[2] Tun PA, Nathan DM, Perlmuter LC (1990) Cognitive and affective disorders in elderly diabetics. *Clin. Geriatr. Med.* 6:731–746.

[3] Arvanitakis Z, Wilson RS, Bienias JL, et al. (2004) Diabetes mellitus and risk of Alzheimer disease and decline in cognitive function. *Arch. Neurol.* 61:661–666. doi: 10.1001/archneur.61.5.661.

[4] Exalto LG, Whitmer RA, Kappele LJ, Biessels GJ (2012) An update on type 2 diabetes, vascular dementia and Alzheimer's disease. *Exp. Gerontol.* 47:858–864. doi: 10.1016/j.exger.2012.07.014.

[5] Mayer G, Nitsch R, Hoyer S (1990) Effects of changes in peripheral and cerebral glucose metabolism on locomotor activity, learning and memory in adult male rats. *Brain Res.* 532:95–100.

[6] Weatherstone K, Meyer T (2012) Streptozocin-based chemotherapy is not history in neuroendocrine tumours. *Target Oncol.* 7:161–168. doi: 10.1007/s11523-012-0224-y.

[7] Lannert H, Hoyer S (1998) Intracerebroventricular administration of streptozotocin causes long-term diminutions in learning and memory abilities and in cerebral energy metabolism in adult rats. *Behav. Neurosci.* 112:1199–1208.

[8] Luo J, Quan J, Tsai J, et al. (1998) Nongenetic mouse models of non-insulin-dependent diabetes mellitus. *Metabolism* 47:663–668.

[9] Schnedl WJ, Ferber S, Johnson JH, Newgard CB (1994) STZ transport and cytotoxicity. Specific enhancement in GLUT2-expressing cells. *Diabetes* 43:1326–1333.

[10] Szkudelski T (2001) The mechanism of alloxan and streptozotocin action in B cells of the rat pancreas. *Physiol. Res. Acad. Sci. Bohemoslov.* 50:537–546.

[11] Reaven GM, Thompson LW, Nahum D, Haskins E (1990) Relationship between hyperglycemia and cognitive function in older NIDDM patients. *Diabetes Care* 13:16–21.

[12] Bjørgaas M, Gimse R, Vik T, Sand T (1997) Cognitive function in type 1 diabetic children with and without episodes of severe hypoglycaemia. *Acta Paediatr. Oslo Nor.* 1992 86:148–153.

[13] Elms SC, Toque HA, Rojas M, et al. (2013) The role of arginase I in diabetes-induced retinal vascular dysfunction in mouse and rat models of diabetes. *Diabetologia* 56:654–662. doi: 10.1007/s00125-012-2789-5.

[14] Sartoretto JL, Oliveira MA, Nigro D, et al. (2007) Constrictor responses to noradrenaline, hemodynamic profile, and superoxide levels measured by hydroethidine oxidation in diabetic rats. *Biol. Pharm. Bull.* 30:1938–1942.

[15] Gispen WH, Biessels GJ (2000) Cognition and synaptic plasticity in diabetes mellitus. *Trends Neurosci.* 23:542–549.

[16] Chabot C, Massicotte G, Milot M, et al. (1997) Impaired modulation of AMPA receptors by calcium-dependent processes in streptozotocin-induced diabetic rats. *Brain Res.* 768:249–256.

[17] Salkovic-Petrisic M, Tribl F, Schmidt M, et al. (2006) Alzheimer-like changes in protein kinase B and glycogen synthase kinase-3 in rat frontal cortex and hippocampus after damage to the insulin signalling pathway. *J. Neurochem.* 96:1005–1015. doi: 10.1111/j.1471-4159.2005.03637.x.

[18] Coleman ES, Dennis JC, Braden TD, et al. (2010) Insulin treatment prevents diabetes-induced alterations in astrocyte glutamate uptake and GFAP content in rats at 4 and 8 weeks of diabetes duration. *Brain Res.* 1306:131–141. doi: 10.1016/j.brainres.2009.10.005.

[19] Revsin Y, Rekers NV, Louwe MC, et al. (2009) Glucocorticoid receptor blockade normalizes hippocampal alterations and cognitive impairment in streptozotocin-induced type 1 diabetes mice. *Neuropsychopharmacol Off. Publ. Am. Coll. Neuropsychopharmacol.* 34:747–758. doi: 10.1038/npp.2008.136.

[20] Gandhi GK, Ball KK, Cruz NF, Dienel GA (2010) Hyperglycaemia and diabetes impair gap junctional communication among astrocytes. *ASN Neuro* 2:e00030. doi: 10.1042/AN20090048.

[21] Zhang T, Pan B-S, Zhao B, et al. (2009) Exacerbation of poststroke dementia by type 2 diabetes is associated with synergistic increases of beta-secretase activation and beta-amyloid generation in rat brains. *Neuroscience* 161:1045–1056. doi: 10.1016/j.neuroscience.2009.04.032.

[22] Van der Heide LP, Ramakers GMJ, Smidt MP (2006) Insulin signaling in the central nervous system: learning to survive. *Prog. Neurobiol.* 79:205–221. doi: 10.1016/j.pneurobio.2006.06.003

[23] Pang ZP, Han W (2012) Regulation of synaptic functions in central nervous system by endocrine hormones and the maintenance of energy homoeostasis. *Biosci. Rep.* 32:423–432. doi: 10.1042/BSR20120026.

[24] Huang X, Wang F, Chen W, et al. (2012) Possible link between the cognitive dysfunction associated with diabetes mellitus and the neurotoxicity of methylglyoxal. *Brain Res.* 1469:82–91. doi: 10.1016/j.brainres.2012.06.011.

[25] Jiang L-Y, Tang S-S, Wang X-Y, et al. (2012) PPARγ agonist pioglitazone reverses memory impairment and biochemical changes in a mouse model of type 2 diabetes mellitus. *CNS Neurosci. Ther.* 18:659–666. doi: 10.1111/j.1755-5949.2012.00341.x.

[26] Daroux M, Prévost G, Maillard-Lefebvre H, et al. (2010) Advanced glycation end-products: implications for diabetic and non-diabetic nephropathies. *Diabetes Metab.* 36:1–10. doi: 10.1016/j.diabet.2009.06.005.

[27] Biessels GJ, van der Heide LP, Kamal A, et al. (2002) Ageing and diabetes: implications for brain function. *Eur. J. Pharmacol.* 441:1–14.

[28] Revsin Y, Saravia F, Roig P, et al. (2005) Neuronal and astroglial alterations in the hippocampus of a mouse model for type 1 diabetes. *Brain Res.* 1038:22–31. doi: 10.1016/j.brainres.2004.12.032.

[29] Wang DD, Bordey A (2008) The astrocyte odyssey. *Prog. Neurobiol.* 86:342–367. doi: 10.1016/j.pneurobio.2008.09.015.

[30] Sofroniew MV, Vinters HV (2010) Astrocytes: biology and pathology. *Acta Neuropathol.* (Berl) 119:7–35. doi: 10.1007/s00401-009-0619-8.

[31] Liberto CM, Albrecht PJ, Herx LM, et al. (2004) Pro-regenerative properties of cytokine-activated astrocytes. *J. Neurochem.* 89:1092–1100. doi: 10.1111/j.1471-4159.2004.02420.x.

[32] Saravia FE, Revsin Y, Gonzalez Deniselle MC, et al. (2002) Increased astrocyte reactivity in the hippocampus of murine models of type 1 diabetes: the nonobese diabetic (NOD) and streptozotocin-treated mice. *Brain Res.* 957:345–353.

[33] Lu M, Xu L, Li B, et al. (2010) Protective effects of grape seed proanthocyanidin extracts on cerebral cortex of streptozotocin-induced diabetic rats through modulating AGEs/RAGE/NF-kappaB pathway. *J. Nutr. Sci. Vitaminol.* (Tokyo) 56:87–97.

[34] Baydas G, Nedzvetskii VS, Tuzcu M, et al. (2003) Increase of glial fibrillary acidic protein and S-100B in hippocampus and cortex of diabetic rats: effects of vitamin E. Eur J Pharmacol 462:67–71.

[35] Baydas G, Reiter RJ, Yasar A, et al. (2003) Melatonin reduces glial reactivity in the hippocampus, cortex, and cerebellum of streptozotocin-induced diabetic rats. *Free Radic Biol. Med.* 35:797–804.

[36] Feit-Leichman RA, Kinouchi R, Takeda M, et al. (2005) Vascular damage in a mouse model of diabetic retinopathy: relation to neuronal and glial changes. *Invest. Ophthalmo.l Vis. Sci.* 46:4281–4287. doi: 10.1167/iovs.04-1361.

[37] Coleman E, Judd R, Hoe L, et al. (2004) Effects of diabetes mellitus on astrocyte GFAP and glutamate transporters in the CNS. *Glia* 48:166–178. doi: 10.1002/glia.20068.

[38] De Senna PN, Ilha J, Baptista PPA, et al. (2011) Effects of physical exercise on spatial memory and astroglial alterations in the hippocampus of diabetic rats. *Metab. Brain Dis.* 26:269–279. doi: 10.1007/s11011-011-9262-x.

[39] Dasuri K, Zhang L, Keller JN (2013) Oxidative stress, neurodegeneration, and the balance of protein degradation and protein synthesis. *Free Radic Biol. Med.* 62:170–185. doi: 10.1016/j.freeradbiomed.2012.09.016.

[40] Allen DA, Yaqoob MM, Harwood SM (2005) Mechanisms of high glucose-induced apoptosis and its relationship to diabetic complications. *J. Nutr. Biochem.* 16:705–713. doi: 10.1016/j.jnutbio.2005.06.007.

[41] Matkovics B, Kotorman M, Varga IS, et al. (1997) Oxidative stress in experimental diabetes induced by streptozotocin. *Acta Physiol. Hung.* 85:29–38.

[42] Mastrocola R, Restivo F, Vercellinatto I, et al. (2005) Oxidative and nitrosative stress in brain mitochondria of diabetic rats. *J. Endocrinol.* 187:37–44. doi: 10.1677/ joe.1.06269.

[43] Kabay SC, Ozden H, Guven G, et al. (2009) Protective effects of vitamin E on central nervous system in streptozotocin-induced diabetic rats. *Clin. Investig. Med. Médecine Clin. Exp.* 32:E314–321.

[44] Kade IJ, Rocha JBT (2013) Gallic acid modulates cerebral oxidative stress conditions and activities of enzyme-dependent signaling systems in streptozotocin-treated rats. *Neurochem. Res.* 38:761–771. doi: 10.1007/s11064-013-0975-6.

[45] Moghaddam HK, Baluchnejadmojarad T, Roghani M, et al. (2013) Berberine Ameliorate Oxidative Stress and Astrogliosis in the Hippocampus of STZ-Induced Diabetic Rats. *Mol. Neurobiol.* doi: 10.1007/s12035-013-8559-7.

[46] Guglielmotto M, Aragno M, Tamagno E, et al. (2012) AGEs/RAGE complex upregulates BACE1 via NF-κB pathway activation. *Neurobiol. Aging* 33:196.e13–27. doi: 10.1016/j.neurobiolaging.2010.05.026.

[47] Liu LP, Hong H, Liao JM, et al. (2009) *Upregulation of RAGE at the blood-brain barrier in streptozotocin-induced diabetic mice.* Synap New York N 63:636–642. doi: 10.1002/syn.20644.

[48] Zong H, Ward M, Madden A, et al. (2010) Hyperglycaemia-induced pro-inflammatory responses by retinal Müller glia are regulated by the receptor for advanced glycation end-products (RAGE). *Diabetologia* 53:2656–2666. doi: 10.1007/ s00125-010-1900-z.

[49] Younessi P, Yoonessi A (2011) Advanced glycation end-products and their receptor-mediated roles: inflammation and oxidative stress. *Iran J. Med. Sci.* 36:154–166.

[50] Havrankova J, Roth J, Brownstein M (1978) Insulin receptors are widely distributed in the central nervous system of the rat. *Nature* 272:827–829.

[51] Pacold ST, Blackard WG (1979) Central nervous system insulin receptors in normal and diabetic rats. *Endocrinology* 105:1452–1457.

[52] Devaskar S, McMenamy K, Holtzclaw L, Sadiq F (1990) Long-term maternal-fetal exposure to high-low insulin concentrations alter liver but not brain insulin receptors. *Am. J. Obstet. Gynecol.* 163:1350–1356.

[53] Pezzino V, Costantino A, Russo P, et al. (1996) Insulin receptor content in tissues of normal and diabetic rats measured by radioimmunoassay. *J. Endocrinol. Invest.* 19: 593–597.

[54] Dou J-T, Chen M, Dufour F, et al. (2005) Insulin receptor signaling in long-term memory consolidation following spatial learning. *Learn Mem. Cold Spring Harb. N* 12:646–655. doi: 10.1101/lm.88005.

[55] Kumar PT, Antony S, Nandhu MS, et al. (2011) Vitamin D3 restores altered cholinergic and insulin receptor expression in the cerebral cortex and muscarinic M3 receptor expression in pancreatic islets of streptozotocin induced diabetic rats. *J. Nutr. Biochem.* 22:418–425. doi: 10.1016/j.jnutbio.2010.03.010.

[56] Peeyush KT, Savitha B, Sherin A, et al. (2010) Cholinergic, dopaminergic and insulin receptors gene expression in the cerebellum of streptozotocin-induced diabetic rats: functional regulation with Vitamin D3 supplementation. *Pharmacol. Biochem. Behav.* 95:216–222. doi: 10.1016/j.pbb.2010.01.008.

[57] Ward MM, Jobling AI, Kalloniatis M, Fletcher EL (2005) Glutamate uptake in retinal glial cells during diabetes. *Diabetologia* 48:351–360. doi: 10.1007/s00125-004-1639-5.

[58] Mehta A, Prabhakar M, Kumar P, et al. (2013) Excitotoxicity: bridge to various triggers in neurodegenerative disorders. *Eur. J. Pharmacol.* 698:6–18. doi: 10.1016/ j.ejphar.2012.10.032.

[59] Matute C, Domercq M, Sánchez-Gómez M-V (2006) Glutamate-mediated glial injury: mechanisms and clinical importance. *Glia* 53:212–224. doi: 10.1002/glia.20275.

[60] Joseph A, Antony S, Paulose CS (2008) Increased glutamate receptor gene expression in the cerebral cortex of insulin induced hypoglycemic and streptozotocin-induced diabetic rats. *Neuroscience* 156:298–304. doi: 10.1016/j.neuroscience. 2008.07.022.

[61] Jayanarayanan S, Smijin S, Peeyush KT, et al. (2013) NMDA and AMPA receptor mediated excitotoxicity in cerebral cortex of streptozotocin induced diabetic rat: ameliorating effects of curcumin. *Chem. Biol. Interact.* 201:39–48. doi: 10.1016/j.cbi. 2012.11.024.

[62] Wasilewska M, Adamiec R (2012) Cerebral regulation of insulin secretion and the development of insulin resistance in type 2 diabetes. *Adv. Clin. Exp. Med. Off. Organ Wroclaw. Med. Univ.* 21:695–703.

[63] Bhardwaj SK, Sandhu SK, Sharma P, Kaur G (1999) Impact of diabetes on CNS: role of signal transduction cascade. *Brain Res. Bull.* 49:155–162.

[64] Sherin A, Anu J, Peeyush KT, et al. (2012) Cholinergic and GABAergic receptor functional deficit in the hippocampus of insulin-induced hypoglycemic and streptozotocin-induced diabetic rats. *Neuroscience* 202:69–76. doi: 10.1016/ j.neuroscience.2011.11.058.

[65] Antony S, Kumar TP, Kuruvilla KP, et al. (2010) Decreased GABA receptor binding in the cerebral cortex of insulin induced hypoglycemic and streptozotocin induced diabetic rats. *Neurochem. Res.* 35:1516–1521. doi: 10.1007/s11064-010-0210-7.

[66] Robinson R, Krishnakumar A, Paulose CS (2009) Enhanced dopamine D1 and D2 receptor gene expression in the hippocampus of hypoglycaemic and diabetic rats. *Cell Mol. Neurobiol.* 29:365–372. doi: 10.1007/s10571-008-9328-4.

[67] Greene DA, Lattimer SA, Sima AA (1987) Sorbitol, phosphoinositides, and sodium-potassium-ATPase in the pathogenesis of diabetic complications. *N. Engl. J. Med.* 316:599–606. doi: 10.1056/NEJM198703053161007.

[68] Leong SF, Leung TK (1991) Diabetes induced by streptozotocin causes reduced Na-K ATPase in the brain. *Neurochem. Res.* 16:1161–1165.

[69] Oner P, Oztaş B, Koçak H (1997) Brain cortex Na(+)-K+ ATPase activities in streptozotocin-diabetic and pentylenetetrazol-epileptic rats. *Pharmacol. Res. Off. J. Ital. Pharmacol. Soc.* 36:69–72. doi: 10.1006/phrs.1997.0208.

[70] Franzon R, Chiarani F, Mendes RH, et al. (2005) Dietary soy prevents brain Na+, K(+)-ATPase reduction in streptozotocin diabetic rats. *Diabetes Res. Clin. Pract.* 69: 107–112. doi: 10.1016/j.diabres.2004.11.010.

[71] Kamboj SS, Chopra K, Sandhir R (2009) Hyperglycemia-induced alterations in synaptosomal membrane fluidity and activity of membrane bound enzymes: beneficial effect of N-acetylcysteine supplementation. *Neuroscience* 162:349–358. doi: 10.1016/ j.neuroscience.2009.05.002.

[72] Faraci FM, Heistad DD (1998) Regulation of the cerebral circulation: role of endothelium and potassium channels. *Physiol. Rev.* 78:53–97.

[73] Minami K, Miki T, Kadowaki T, Seino S (2004) Roles of ATP-sensitive K+ channels as metabolic sensors: studies of Kir6.x null mice. *Diabetes* 53 Suppl 3:S176–180.

[74] Heng L-J, Yang R-H, Jia D (2011) Diabetes impairs learning performance through affecting membrane excitability of hippocampal pyramidal neurons. *Behav. Brain Res.* 224:250–258. doi: 10.1016/j.bbr.2011.05.043.

[75] Gonçalves C-A, Leite MC, Nardin P (2008) Biological and methodological features of the measurement of S100B, a putative marker of brain injury. *Clin. Biochem.* 41: 755–763. doi: 10.1016/j.clinbiochem.2008.04.003.

[76] Donato R (2003) Intracellular and extracellular roles of S100 proteins. *Microsc. Res. Tech.* 60:540–551. doi: 10.1002/jemt.10296.

[77] Donato R, Sorci G, Riuzzi F, et al. (2009) S100B's double life: intracellular regulator and extracellular signal. *Biochim. Biophys. Acta* 1793:1008–1022. doi: 10.1016/j.bbamcr.2008.11.009.

[78] Ostendorp T, Leclerc E, Galichet A, et al. (2007) Structural and functional insights into RAGE activation by multimeric S100B. *EMBO J.* 26:3868–3878. doi: 10.1038/sj.emboj.7601805.

[79] Ponath G, Schettler C, Kaestner F, et al. (2007) Autocrine S100B effects on astrocytes are mediated via RAGE. *J. Neuroimmunol.* 184:214–222. doi: 10.1016/ j.jneuroim.2006.12.011.

[80] Van Eldik LJ, Wainwright MS (2003) The Janus face of glial-derived S100B: beneficial and detrimental functions in the brain. *Restor. Neurol. Neurosci.* 21:97–108.

[81] Michetti F, Corvino V, Geloso MC, et al. (2012) The S100B protein in biological fluids: more than a lifelong biomarker of brain distress. *J. Neurochem.* 120:644–659. doi: 10.1111/j.1471-4159.2011.07612.x.

[82] Berger RP, Beers SR, Richichi R, et al. (2007) Serum biomarker concentrations and outcome after pediatric traumatic brain injury. *J. Neurotrauma* 24:1793–1801. doi: 10.1089/neu.2007.0316.

[83] Tanaka Y, Marumo T, Omura T, Yoshida S (2008) Relationship between cerebrospinal and peripheral S100B levels after focal cerebral ischemia in rats. *Neurosci. Lett.* 436:40–43. doi: 10.1016/j.neulet.2008.02.056.

[84] Schroeter ML, Sacher J, Steiner J, et al. (2013) Serum S100B represents a new biomarker for mood disorders. *Curr. Drug Targets* 14:1237–1248.

[85] Steiner J, Bogerts B, Schroeter ML, Bernstein H-G (2011) S100B protein in neurodegenerative disorders. *Clin. Chem. Lab. Med. CCLM FESCC* 49:409–424. doi: 10.1515/CCLM.2011.083.

[86] Chaves ML, Camozzato AL, Ferreira ED, et al. (2010) Serum levels of S100B and NSE proteins in Alzheimer's disease patients. *J. Neuroinflammation* 7:6. doi: 10.1186/ 1742-2094-7-6.

[87] Gonçalves CA, Leite MC, Guerra MC (2010) Adipocytes as an Important Source of Serum S100B and Possible Roles of This Protein in Adipose Tissue. *Cardiovasc. Psychiatry Neurol.* 2010:790431. doi: 10.1155/2010/790431.

[88] Hovsepyan MR, Haas MJ, Boyajyan AS, et al. (2004) Astrocytic and neuronal biochemical markers in the sera of subjects with diabetes mellitus. *Neurosci. Lett.* 369: 224–227. doi: 10.1016/j.neulet.2004.07.071.

[89] Penfold SA, Coughlan MT, Patel SK, et al. (2010) Circulating high-molecular-weight RAGE ligands activate pathways implicated in the development of diabetic nephropathy. *Kidney Int.* 78:287–295. doi: 10.1038/ki.2010.134.

[90] Shanmugam N, Todorov IT, Nair I, et al. (2006) Increased expression of cyclooxygenase-2 in human pancreatic islets treated with high glucose or ligands of the advanced glycation endproduct-specific receptor (AGER), and in islets from diabetic mice. *Diabetologia* 49:100–107. doi: 10.1007/s00125-005-0065-7.

[91] Reddy MA, Li S-L, Sahar S, et al. (2006) Key role of Src kinase in S100B-induced activation of the receptor for advanced glycation end products in vascular smooth muscle cells. *J. Biol. Chem.* 281:13685–13693. doi: 10.1074/jbc.M511425200.

[92] Zimmer DB, Chessher J, Wilson GL, Zimmer WE (1997) S100A1 and S100B expression and target proteins in type I diabetes. *Endocrinology* 138:5176–5183.

[93] Nardin P, Tramontina F, Leite MC, et al. (2007) S100B content and secretion decrease in astrocytes cultured in high-glucose medium. *Neurochem. Int.* 50:774–782. doi: 10.1016/j.neuint.2007.01.013.

[94] Querfurth HW, LaFerla FM (2010) Alzheimer's disease. *N. Engl. J. Med.* 362:329–344. doi: 10.1056/NEJMra0909142.

[95] Candore G, Bulati M, Caruso C, et al. (2010) Inflammation, cytokines, immune response, apolipoprotein E, cholesterol, and oxidative stress in Alzheimer disease: therapeutic implications. *Rejuvenation Res.* 13:301–313. doi: 10.1089/rej.2009.0993.

[96] Selkoe DJ (2002) Alzheimer's disease is a synaptic failure. *Science* 298:789–791. doi: 10.1126/science.1074069.

[97] Mattson MP, Chan SL (2003) Neuronal and glial calcium signaling in Alzheimer's disease. *Cell Calcium* 34:385–397.

[98] Correia SC, Santos RX, Perry G, et al. (2011) Insulin-resistant brain state: the culprit in sporadic Alzheimer's disease? *Ageing Res. Rev.* 10:264–273. doi: 10.1016/ j.arr.2011.01.001.

[99] De la Monte SM, Wands JR (2008) Alzheimer's disease is type 3 diabetes-evidence reviewed. *J. Diabetes Sci. Technol.* 2:1101–1113.

[100] Simpson IA, Chundu KR, Davies-Hill T, et al. (1994) Decreased concentrations of GLUT1 and GLUT3 glucose transporters in the brains of patients with Alzheimer's disease. *Ann. Neurol.* 35:546–551. doi: 10.1002/ana.410350507.

[101] Gibson GE, Sheu KF, Blass JP, et al. (1988) Reduced activities of thiamine-dependent enzymes in the brains and peripheral tissues of patients with Alzheimer's disease. *Arch. Neurol.* 45:836–840.

[102] Mastrogiacoma F, Bettendorff L, Grisar T, Kish SJ (1996) Brain thiamine, its phosphate esters, and its metabolizing enzymes in Alzheimer's disease. *Ann. Neurol.* 39:585–591. doi: 10.1002/ana.410390507.

[103] Mattson MP, Gary DS, Chan SL, Duan W (2001) Perturbed endoplasmic reticulum function, synaptic apoptosis and the pathogenesis of Alzheimer's disease. *Biochem. Soc. Symp.* 151–162.

[104] Frölich L, Blum-Degen D, Bernstein HG, et al. (1998) Brain insulin and insulin receptors in aging and sporadic Alzheimer's disease. *J. Neural. Transm. Vienna Austria* 1996 105:423–438.

[105] Lester-Coll N, Rivera EJ, Soscia SJ, et al. (2006) Intracerebral streptozotocin model of type 3 diabetes: relevance to sporadic Alzheimer's disease. *J. Alzheimers Dis. JAD* 9:13–33.

[106] Rivera EJ, Goldin A, Fulmer N, et al. (2005) Insulin and insulin-like growth factor expression and function deteriorate with progression of Alzheimer's disease: link to brain reductions in acetylcholine. *J. Alzheimers Dis. JAD* 8:247–268.

[107] Watson GS, Craft S (2004) Modulation of memory by insulin and glucose: neuropsychological observations in Alzheimer's disease. *Eur. J. Pharmacol.* 490:97–113. doi: 10.1016/j.ejphar.2004.02.048.

[108] Sharma M, Gupta YK (2001) Intracerebroventricular injection of streptozotocin in rats produces both oxidative stress in the brain and cognitive impairment. *Life Sci.* 68:1021–1029.

[109] Mayer, G., Nitsch, R., Hoyer, S. (1989) Impairments in passive avoidance learning after cerebral inhibition of cerebral glucose metabolism. *J. Neural. Transm. 1 Park Dis. Dement. Sect.* 103–104.

[110] Hellweg R, Nitsch R, Hock C, et al. (1992) Nerve growth factor and choline acetyltransferase activity levels in the rat brain following experimental impairment of cerebral glucose and energy metabolism. *J. Neurosci. Res.* 31:479–486. doi: 10.1002/jnr.490310310.

[111] Rodrigues L, Dutra MF, Ilha J, et al. (2010) Treadmill training restores spatial cognitive deficits and neurochemical alterations in the hippocampus of rats submitted to an intracerebroventricular administration of streptozotocin. *J. Neural. Transm. Vienna Austria* 1996 117:1295–1305. doi: 10.1007/s00702-010-0501-9.

[112] Sharma M, Gupta YK (2002) Chronic treatment with trans resveratrol prevents intracerebroventricular streptozotocin induced cognitive impairment and oxidative stress in rats. *Life Sci.* 71:2489–2498.

[113] Tramontina AC, Wartchow KM, Rodrigues L, et al. (2011) The neuroprotective effect of two statins: simvastatin and pravastatin on a streptozotocin-induced model of Alzheimer's disease in rats. *J. Neural. Transm. Vienna Austria* 1996 118:1641–1649. doi: 10.1007/s00702-011-0680-z.

[114] Duelli R, Schröck H, Kuschinsky W, Hoyer S (1994) Intracerebroventricular injection of streptozotocin induces discrete local changes in cerebral glucose utilization in rats. *Int. J. Dev. Neurosci. Off. J. Int. Soc. Dev. Neurosci.* 12:737–743.

[115] Pathan AR, Viswanad B, Sonkusare SK, Ramarao P (2006) Chronic administration of pioglitazone attenuates intracerebroventricular streptozotocin induced-memory impairment in rats. *Life Sci.* 79:2209–2216. doi: 10.1016/j.lfs.2006.07.018.

[116] Plaschke K, Hoyer S (1993) Action of the diabetogenic drug streptozotocin on glycolytic and glycogenolytic metabolism in adult rat brain cortex and hippocampus. *Int. J. Dev. Neurosci. Off. J. Int. Soc. Dev. Neurosci.* 11:477–483.

[117] Nitsch R, Hoyer S (1991) Local action of the diabetogenic drug, streptozotocin, on glucose and energy metabolism in rat brain cortex. *Neurosci. Lett.* 128:199–202.

[118] Gerozissis K (2008) Brain insulin, energy and glucose homeostasis; genes, environment and metabolic pathologies. *Eur. J. Pharmacol.* 585:38–49. doi: 10.1016/j.ejphar.2008.01.050.

[119] Baki L, Neve RL, Shao Z, et al. (2008) Wild-type but not FAD mutant presenilin-1 prevents neuronal degeneration by promoting phosphatidylinositol 3-kinase neuroprotective signaling. *J. Neurosci. Off. J. Soc. Neurosci.* 28:483–490. doi: 10.1523/JNEUROSCI.4067-07.2008.

[120] Gasparini L, Netzer WJ, Greengard P, Xu H (2002) Does insulin dysfunction play a role in Alzheimer's disease? *Trends Pharmacol. Sci.* 23:288–293.

[121] Steen E, Terry BM, Rivera EJ, et al. (2005) Impaired insulin and insulin-like growth factor expression and signaling mechanisms in Alzheimer's disease--is this type 3 diabetes? *J. Alzheimers Dis. JAD* 7:63–80.

[122] Grünblatt E, Salkovic-Petrisic M, Osmanovic J, et al. (2007) Brain insulin system dysfunction in streptozotocin intracerebroventricularly treated rats generates hyperphosphorylated tau protein. *J. Neurochem.* 101:757–770. doi: 10.1111/j.1471-4159.2006.04368.x.

[123] Deng Y, Li B, Liu Y, et al. (2009) Dysregulation of insulin signaling, glucose transporters, O-GlcNAcylation, and phosphorylation of tau and neurofilaments in the brain: Implication for Alzheimer's disease. *Am. J. Pathol.* 175:2089–2098. doi: 10.2353/ajpath.2009.090157.

[124] De la Monte SM, Tong M, Lester-Coll N, et al. (2006) Therapeutic rescue of neurodegeneration in experimental type 3 diabetes: relevance to Alzheimer's disease. *J Alzheimers Dis. JAD* 10:89–109.

[125] Ferrer I, Gomez-Isla T, Puig B, et al. (2005) Current advances on different kinases involved in tau phosphorylation, and implications in Alzheimer's disease and tauopathies. *Curr. Alzheimer Res.* 2:3–18.

[126] Xiong H, Zheng C, Wang J, et al. (2013) The neuroprotection of liraglutide on Alzheimer-like learning and memory impairment by modulating the hyperphosphorylation of tau and neurofilament proteins and insulin signaling pathways in mice. *J. Alzheimers Dis. JAD* 37:623–635. doi: 10.3233/JAD-130584.

[127] Zhou S, Yu G, Chi L, et al. (2013) Neuroprotective effects of edaravone on cognitive deficit, oxidative stress and tau hyperphosphorylation induced by intracerebroventricular streptozotocin in rats. *Neurotoxicology* 38:136–145. doi: 10.1016/j.neuro.2013.07.007.

[128] Ke YD, Delerue F, Gladbach A, et al. (2009) Experimental diabetes mellitus exacerbates tau pathology in a transgenic mouse model of Alzheimer's disease. *PloS One* 4:e7917. doi: 10.1371/journal.pone.0007917.

[129] Plaschke K, Kopitz J, Siegelin M, et al. (2010) Insulin-resistant brain state after intracerebroventricular streptozotocin injection exacerbates Alzheimer-like changes in Tg2576 AbetaPP-overexpressing mice. *J. Alzheimers Dis. JAD* 19:691–704. doi: 10.3233/JAD-2010-1270.

[130] Salkovic-Petrisic M, Knezovic A, Hoyer S, Riederer P (2013) What have we learned from the streptozotocin-induced animal model of sporadic Alzheimer's disease, about the therapeutic strategies in Alzheimer's research. *J. Neural. Transm. Vienna Austria* 1996 120:233–252. doi: 10.1007/s00702-012-0877-9.

[131] Ishrat T, Khan MB, Hoda MN, et al. (2006) Coenzyme Q10 modulates cognitive impairment against intracerebroventricular injection of streptozotocin in rats. *Behav. Brain Res.* 171:9–16. doi: 10.1016/j.bbr.2006.03.009.

[132] Prickaerts J, Fahrig T, Blokland A (1999) Cognitive performance and biochemical markers in septum, hippocampus and striatum of rats after an i.c.v. injection of streptozotocin: a correlation analysis. *Behav. Brain Res.* 102:73–88.

[133] Biasibetti R, Tramontina AC, Costa AP, et al. (2013) Green tea (-)epigallocatechin-3-gallate reverses oxidative stress and reduces acetylcholinesterase activity in a

streptozotocin-induced model of dementia. *Behav. Brain Res.* 236:186–193. doi: 10.1016/j.bbr.2012.08.039.

[134] Sodhi RK, Singh N (2013) Defensive effect of lansoprazole in dementia of AD type in mice exposed to streptozotocin and cholesterol enriched diet. *PloS One* 8:e70487. doi: 10.1371/journal.pone.0070487.

[135] Paula-Lima AC, Brito-Moreira J, Ferreira ST (2013) Deregulation of excitatory neurotransmission underlying synapse failure in Alzheimer's disease. *J. Neurochem.* 126:191–202. doi: 10.1111/jnc.12304

[136] Robinson SR (2001) Changes in the cellular distribution of glutamine synthetase in Alzheimer's disease. *J. Neurosci. Res.* 66:972–980.

[137] Verkhratsky A, Olabarria M, Noristani HN, et al. (2010) Astrocytes in Alzheimer's disease. *Neurother. J. Am. Soc. Exp. Neurother.* 7:399–412. doi: 10.1016/j.nurt.2010.05.017.

[138] Van Eldik LJ, Griffin WS (1994) S100 beta expression in Alzheimer's disease: relation to neuropathology in brain regions. *Biochim. Biophys. Acta* 1223:398–403.

[139] Nagele RG, Wegiel J, Venkataraman V, et al. (2004) Contribution of glial cells to the development of amyloid plaques in Alzheimer's disease. *Neurobiol. Aging* 25:663–674. doi: 10.1016/j.neurobiolaging.2004.01.007.

[140] Sheng JG, Mrak RE, Bales KR, et al. (2000) Overexpression of the neuritotrophic cytokine S100beta precedes the appearance of neuritic beta-amyloid plaques in APPV717F mice. *J. Neurochem.* 74:295–301.

[141] Mori T, Koyama N, Arendash GW, et al. (2010) Overexpression of human S100B exacerbates cerebral amyloidosis and gliosis in the Tg2576 mouse model of Alzheimer's disease. *Glia* 58:300–314. doi: 10.1002/glia.20924.

[142] Rothermundt M, Peters M, Prehn JHM, Arolt V (2003) S100B in brain damage and neurodegeneration. *Microsc. Res. Tech.* 60:614–632. doi: 10.1002/jemt.10303.

[143] Hosseinzadeh S, Zahmatkesh M, Zarrindast M-R, et al. (2013) Elevated CSF and plasma microparticles in a rat model of streptozotocin-induced cognitive impairment. *Behav. Brain Res.* 256:503–511. doi: 10.1016/j.bbr.2013.09.019.

[144] Vicente E, Degerone D, Bohn L, et al. (2009) Astroglial and cognitive effects of chronic cerebral hypoperfusion in the rat. *Brain Res.* 1251:204–212. doi: 10.1016/j.brainres.2008.11.032.

[145] Costa AP, Tramontina AC, Biasibetti R, et al. (2012) Neuroglial alterations in rats submitted to the okadaic acid-induced model of dementia. *Behav. Brain Res.* 226:420–427. doi: 10.1016/j.bbr.2011.09.035.

[146] Weinstock M, Shoham S (2004) Rat models of dementia based on reductions in regional glucose metabolism, cerebral blood flow and cytochrome oxidase activity. *J. Neural. Transm. Vienna Austria* 1996 111:347–366. doi: 10.1007/s00702-003-0058-y.

[147] Chen Y, Liang Z, Blanchard J, et al. (2013) A non-transgenic mouse model (icv-STZ mouse) of Alzheimer's disease: similarities to and differences from the transgenic model (3xTg-AD mouse). *Mol. Neurobiol.* 47:711–725. doi: 10.1007/s12035-012-8375-5.

[148] Pellerin L, Magistretti PJ (1994) Glutamate uptake into astrocytes stimulates aerobic glycolysis: a mechanism coupling neuronal activity to glucose utilization. *Proc. Natl. Acad. Sci. U S A* 91:10625–10629.

[149] Guzmán M, Blázquez C (2001) Is there an astrocyte-neuron ketone body shuttle? *Trends Endocrinol. Metab. TEM* 12:169–173.

[150] Pfrieger FW, Ungerer N (2011) Cholesterol metabolism in neurons and astrocytes. *Prog. Lipid Res.* 50:357–371. doi: 10.1016/j.plipres.2011.06.002.

[151] Dringen R, Hirrlinger J (2003) Glutathione pathways in the brain. *Biol. Chem.* 384: 505–516. doi: 10.1515/BC.2003.059.

[152] Cooper AJL (2012) The role of glutamine synthetase and glutamate dehydrogenase in cerebral ammonia homeostasis. *Neurochem. Res.* 37:2439–2455. doi: 10.1007/s11064-012-0803-4.

[153] Schousboe A, Bak LK, Waagepetersen HS (2013) Astrocytic Control of Biosynthesis and Turnover of the Neurotransmitters Glutamate and GABA. *Front Endocrinol.* 4:102. doi: 10.3389/fendo.2013.00102.

[154] Townsend M, Mehta T, Selkoe DJ (2007) Soluble Abeta inhibits specific signal transduction cascades common to the insulin receptor pathway. *J. Biol. Chem.* 282: 33305–33312. doi: 10.1074/jbc.M610390200.

[155] Grodstein F, Chen J, Wilson RS, et al. (2001) Type 2 diabetes and cognitive function in community-dwelling elderly women. *Diabetes Care* 24:1060–1065.

[156] Park SA (2011) A common pathogenic mechanism linking type-2 diabetes and Alzheimer's disease: evidence from animal models. *J. Clin. Neurol. Seoul Korea* 7:10–18. doi: 10.3988/jcn.2011.7.1.10.

[157] Reitz C (2012) Alzheimer's disease and the amyloid cascade hypothesis: a critical review. *Int. J. Alzheimers Dis.* 2012:369808. doi: 10.1155/2012/369808.

[158] Chen Z, Zhong C (2013) Decoding Alzheimer's disease from perturbed cerebral glucose metabolism: implications for diagnostic and therapeutic strategies. *Prog. Neurobiol.* 108:21–43. doi: 10.1016/j.pneurobio.2013.06.004.

[159] Mosconi L, De Santi S, Li Y, et al. (2006) Visual rating of medial temporal lobe metabolism in mild cognitive impairment and Alzheimer's disease using FDG-PET. *Eur. J. Nucl. Med. Mol. Imaging* 33:210–221. doi: 10.1007/s00259-005-1956-z.

[160] Cunnane S, Nugent S, Roy M, et al. (2011) Brain fuel metabolism, aging, and Alzheimer's disease. *Nutr. Burbank Los Angeles Cty Calif.* 27:3–20. doi: 10.1016/j.nut.2010.07.021.

[161] Jakobsen J, Nedergaard M, Aarslew-Jensen M, Diemer NH (1990) Regional brain glucose metabolism and blood flow in streptozocin-induced diabetic rats. *Diabetes* 39:437–440.

[162] Heo J-H, Lee S-R, Lee S-T, et al. (2011) Spatial distribution of glucose hypometabolism induced by intracerebroventricular streptozotocin in monkeys. *J. Alzheimers Dis. JAD* 25:517–523. doi: 10.3233/JAD-2011-102079.

[163] Cardoso S, Santos RX, Correia SC, et al. (2012) Insulin-induced recurrent hypoglycemia exacerbates diabetic brain mitochondrial dysfunction and oxidative imbalance. *Neurobiol. Dis.* 49C:1–12. doi: 10.1016/j.nbd.2012.08.008.

[164] Pekny M, Pekna M (2004) Astrocyte intermediate filaments in CNS pathologies and regeneration. *J. Pathol.* 204:428–437. doi: 10.1002/path.1645.

[165] Saxena G, Patro IK, Nath C (2011) ICV STZ induced impairment in memory and neuronal mitochondrial function: A protective role of nicotinic receptor. *Behav. Brain Res.* 224:50–57. doi: 10.1016/j.bbr.2011.04.039.

[166] Zhou Y, Qu Z, Zeng Y, et al. (2012) Neuroprotective effect of preadministration with Ganoderma lucidum spore on rat hippocampus. *Exp. Toxicol. Pathol. Off. J. Ges. Für Toxikol. Pathol.* 64:673–680. doi: 10.1016/j.etp.2010.12.011.
[167] Thorens B (1996) Glucose transporters in the regulation of intestinal, renal, and liver glucose fluxes. *Am. J. Physiol.* 270:G541–553.
[168] Unger RH (1991) Diabetic hyperglycemia: link to impaired glucose transport in pancreatic beta cells. *Science* 251:1200–1205.
[169] Brant AM, Jess TJ, Milligan G, et al. (1993) Immunological analysis of glucose transporters expressed in different regions of the rat brain and central nervous system. *Biochem. Biophys. Res. Commun.* 192:1297–1302. doi: 10.1006/bbrc.1993.1557.
[170] Navarro M, Rodriquez de Fonseca F, Alvarez E, et al. (1996) Colocalization of glucagon-like peptide-1 (GLP-1) receptors, glucose transporter GLUT-2, and glucokinase mRNAs in rat hypothalamic cells: evidence for a role of GLP-1 receptor agonists as an inhibitory signal for food and water intake. *J. Neurochem.* 67:1982–1991.
[171] Rodríguez EM, Blázquez JL, Pastor FE, et al. (2005) Hypothalamic tanycytes: a key component of brain-endocrine interaction. *Int. Rev. Cytol.* 247:89–164. doi: 10.1016/S0074-7696(05)47003-5.
[172] Leloup C, Arluison M, Lepetit N, et al. (1994) Glucose transporter 2 (GLUT 2): expression in specific brain nuclei. *Brain Res.* 638:221–226.
[173] Baydas G, Sonkaya E, Tuzcu M, et al. (2005) Novel role for gabapentin in neuroprotection of central nervous system in streptozotocine-induced diabetic rats. *Acta Pharmacol. Sin.* 26:417–422. doi: 10.1111/j.1745-7254.2005.00072.x.
[174] Dennis JC, Coleman ES, Swyers SE, et al. (2005) Changes in mitotic rate and GFAP expression in the primary olfactory axis of streptozotocin-induced diabetic rats. *J. Neurocytol.* 34:3–10. doi: 10.1007/s11068-005-5044-x.
[175] Lebed YV, Orlovsky MA, Nikonenko AG, et al. (2008) Early reaction of astroglial cells in rat hippocampus to streptozotocin-induced diabetes. *Neurosci. Lett.* 444:181–185. doi: 10.1016/j.neulet.2008.07.094.
[176] Collino M, Aragno M, Castiglia S, et al. (2009) Insulin reduces cerebral ischemia/reperfusion injury in the hippocampus of diabetic rats: a role for glycogen synthase kinase-3beta. *Diabetes* 58:235–242. doi: 10.2337/db08-0691.
[177] Rodrigues L, Biasibetti R, Swarowsky A, et al. (2009) Hippocampal alterations in rats submitted to streptozotocin-induced dementia model are prevented by aminoguanidine. *J. Alzheimers Dis. JAD* 17:193–202. doi: 10.3233/JAD-2009-1034.
[178] Muller AP, Zimmer ER, Kalinine E, et al. (2012) Physical exercise exacerbates memory deficits induced by intracerebroventricular STZ but improves insulin regulation of $H_2O_2$ production in mice synaptosomes. *J. Alzheimers Dis. JAD* 30: 889–898. doi: 10.3233/JAD-2012-112066.

In: Streptozotocin: Uses, Mechanism of Action and Side Effects ISBN: 978-1-63117-255-7
Editor: Elizabeth L. Gauthier 

*Chapter 4*

# STREPTOZOTOCIN-INDUCED RODENT MODELS OF DIABETES: PROTOCOL COMPARISONS

***Renata O. Samuel, João E. Gomes-Filho, Eloi Dezan-Júnior and Luciano T. A. Cintra****

Faculdade de Odontologia de Araçatuba, UNESP Univ Estadual Paulista, Departamento de Odontologia Restauradora, Araçatuba, São Paulo, Brazil

## ABSTRACT

Type 1 and type 2 diabetes mellitus (DM) are characterized by hyperglycemia, due to lost or damaged insulin-producing β-cells within the pancreatic islets of Langerhans. Rodent models of DM result in hyperglycemia, arising from different forms of islet deterioration. Streptozotocin (STZ) is currently used to induce experimental DM in rodents because it selectively targets pancreatic β-cells. STZ enters β-cells via a glucose transporter (GLUT2), causing DNA alkylation, which in turn activates poly ADP-ribosylation, leading to ATP depletion and resulting in the formation of superoxide anions. Concomitantly, STZ triggers nitric oxide formation, which results in DNA damage. Both of these actions cause β-cell necrosis, leading to DM. These features provide a methodological advantage for STZ, resulting in the development of human-like DM. However, there is no consensus across the literature regarding the optimal STZ dose or administration route for developing rodent models of DM. In addition, the nutritional status of the animals employed has also been shown to influence outcomes. This review aims to compare the different methodologies, considering their advantages and disadvantages.

**Keywords:** Streptozotocin, Rodent models, rat, mice

* Corresponding author: Luciano T. A. Cintra, Faculdade de Odontologia de Araçatuba, UNESP Univ Estadual Paulista, Departamento de Odontologia Restauradora, R. José Bonifacio, 1193 Araçatuba- São Paulo, Brazil. Tel.: +(0055) 18 36362867, Fax: +(0055) 18 36363253, E-mail: lucianocintra@foa.unesp.br.

# UNIT 1 – STREPTOZOTOCIN CHARACTERISTICS

## 1.1. History

STZ is a compound that was originally identified in the late 1950s as an antibiotic, produced by Streptomyces achromogenes [1]. Its molecular structure (Figure 1) corresponds to a 2-deoxy-d-glucose molecule substituted at C2 with a N-methyl-N-nitrosourea group [2]. It has been synthesized using three different procedures: i) from tetra-O-acetyl glucosamine hydrochloride [2]; ii) from d-glucosamine + N-nitrosomethyl carbamyl-azide [3] and iii) from d-glucosamine N-methylurea [4].

In the late 1960s came the first reports of STZ as an antineoplastic agent [5-7]. Although it can still be used for cancer therapy, the genotoxic effects of STZ render it highly mutagenic, causing DNA and chromosome damage by free radicals generated during STZ metabolism [8].

The genotoxic effects of STZ on pancreatic β-cells have been useful for inducing insulitis and DM in experimental animals [9]. This approach to producing animal models of DM has been shown to be dependable and is commonly used in scientific research [10–12].

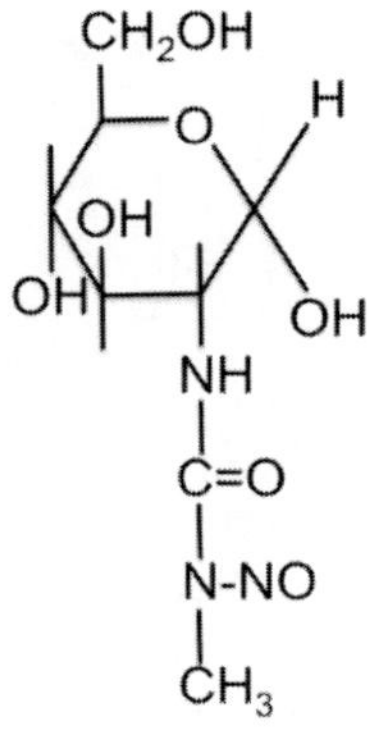


Figure 1. Structure of STZ [2].

## 1.2. Diabetogenic Effects of STZ

STZ can be used to induce both insulin-dependent and non-insulin-dependent DM. As STZ is an analogue of N-acetylglucosamine, it can enter the β-cells via a cell membrane glucose transporter (GLUT2). STZ causes alkylation of DNA, an activity related to its nitrosourea moiety, especially at the O6 position of guanine [13].

The diabetogenic effects of STZ correlate with the activation of poly ADP-ribosylation, which reduces ATP, NAD and NADH levels in the pancreatic β-cells [14], causing inhibition of insulin synthesis and secretion [15]. Moreover, STZ removed the ability of the cells to generate action potentials when stimulated by D-glucose, D-mannose, L-leucine, or D-glyceraldehyde, substances that are known to evoke insulin secretion [16].

The high concentration of intracellular ADP in STZ-treated cells results in increased ADP degradation to produce hypoxanthine, a substrate of xanthine oxidase (XO), which is highly active in β-cells [17]. XO uses molecular oxygen as an electron acceptor, producing hydrogen peroxide and superoxide anion. Therefore, XO can act as an important biological source of reactive oxygen species [18].

Elevated levels of nitric oxide (NO) in STZ-treated cells also contribute to STZ-induced DNA damage [19, 20]. This excess NO production results from a STZ-induced increase in NO synthase (NOS) activity. Thus, this compound produces an imbalance between the levels of reactive oxygen species and the related cellular defense mechanisms, resulting in tissue injury [21, 22].

Superoxide dismutase is a widely distributed enzyme that scavenges superoxide radicals. It is primarily located in the cytosol and mitochondria of cells. Previous studies showed that diabetogenic drugs may exert their cytotoxic effects in part by inhibiting superoxide dismutase [23]. In conclusion, STZ has three main diabetogenic effects: i) alkylation of DNA [13], ii) formation of superoxide radicals [17, 21, 22]; and iii) inhibition of superoxide dismutase [23] (Figure 2).

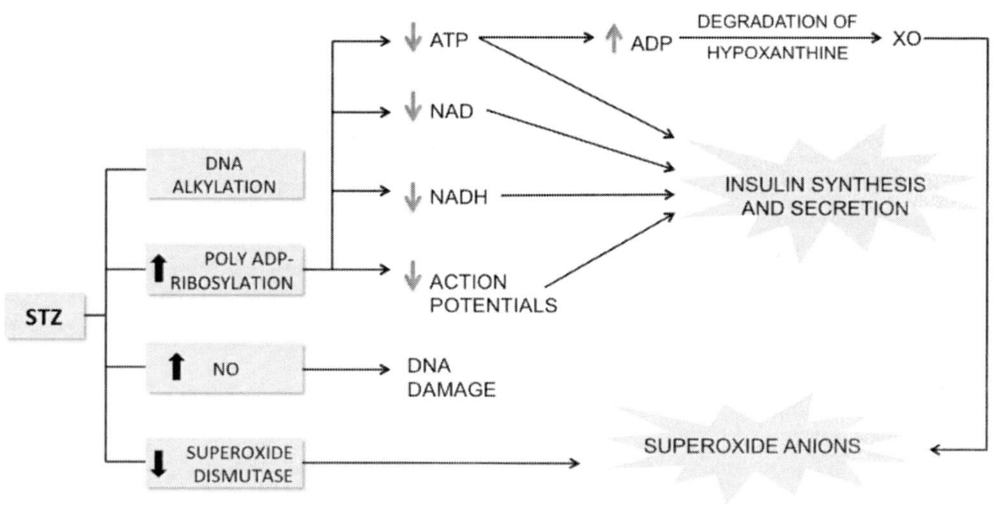


Figure 2. Demonstration of the main diabetogenic activities of STZ.

## 1.3. Side Effects of STZ

Most research employing STZ in rodents has focused on its diabetogenic properties, rather than its side effects. However, STZ has also been reported to be mutagenic and carcinogenic [24-28]. These genotoxic effects arise from the generation of superoxides, peroxinitrates, hydroxyl radicals, and hydrogen peroxide [8, 29, 30]. In addition, STZ is a potent alkylating agent, known to directly methylate DNA [31], as well as inducing DNA strand breaks and alkali-labile sites [32, 33].

Many studies have reported the presence of cancer in rodents treated with STZ [24, 34–36]. This tumorigenic activity of STZ can be enhanced when it is co-administered with certain drugs, such as nicotinamide [35, 37]. Although some researchers consider that administration of STZ and nicotinamide produces an ideal rodent model of DM [35, 37], the potential side effects of this combination have not been studied thoroughly in rodents.

The genotoxicity of STZ may be age dependent, producing greater effects on younger animals [38]. A study reported that the frequency of bone marrow micronucleated cells in animals treated with STZ was age dependent, and that there was a higher frequency of micronucleated polychromatic erythrocytes in neonatal and young rats than in adults [39]. This may be due to the higher rate of cell proliferation and respiration in the target cells of neonatal and young rats [39]. The extent of DNA damage and cellular proliferation in rat kidneys, and the time course of repair, have been studied following single doses of STZ (0.25–60 mg/kg) [40].

This study reported that 2.5 mg/kg STZ was the lowest dose found to induce detectable DNA strand breaks. Extensive DNA damage was produced by the commonly used diabetogenic dose of 60 mg/kg and was still detectable 3–9 days after dosing. Levels of damage had returned to near background levels by 27 days after treatment with 60 mg/kg STZ. These findings led the authors to propose that there should be a delay between administration of STZ and testing of potential experimental therapies in this model, to avoid potential additive or synergistic effects on STZ-induced nephrotoxicity and/or genotoxicity [40]. However, this is not commonly practiced, as the experimental phase of such studies is usually initiated upon confirmation of hyperglycemia. It was recently proposed that a high-fat diet influenced the effects of STZ in rodents. However, it is not known whether this improves or worsens the genotoxicity of STZ and further studies are required to elucidate this.

# UNIT 2 – THE RODENT MODELS

## 2.1. Experimentally Induced Models of DM

Animal models should be used to study specific genotypic or phenotypic aspects of DM, rather than assuming that a single animal model can accurately reflect the diverse manifestations of the human disease [41]. An extensive range of mammalian models has been developed, including non-human primates, pigs, dogs, cats, rabbits, rats, and mice [42]. There are many variables to consider when comparing animal models, including whether animals are fasted prior to STZ administration, age of animals, strain, STZ dose, administration route, drug interactions, and side effects.

The ability of animal models to achieve a pathological state that has clinical relevance depends on the establishment of a consistent level of glycemia for the duration of the experiment [43]. The development of a consensus around the optimal protocols for establishing and analyzing STZ-induced diabetic models would greatly facilitate rational comparison of these [43].

Rodent models are generally preferred due to their smaller body size, omnivorous nature, and tranquil behavior, features that reduce dietary and housing costs and facilitate handling by researchers [42]. However, the protocols for induction of DM in rodent models with STZ are highly variable. There are three approaches described in literature: i) the injection of small doses of STZ on consecutive days, ii) the injection of a single high dose of STZ, and iii) the administration of small doses or single dose of STZ in conjunction with a high-fat diet. In this review, we will consider the advantages and disadvantages of these rodent models, and discuss their variability in the literature.

## 2.2. Animal Strains Used for STZ DM Models

Albino Wistar and Sprague-Dawley rat strains are among the most commonly used rodents for STZ-induced models of DM. Both are widely used in published models and have contributed greatly to scientific research [44-48]. Other strains have also shown promising responses, such as nude mice [49], Zucker fatty rats [50], and C57BL/6J mice [51], among others [52].

There are no recommendations in the literature regarding the strain of rodent producing the best DM model. However, one study emphasized the importance of exploratory safety assessments when selecting a nude mouse source [49]. Although each rodent strain generally has the same origin, each vendor provides a unique subline [49].

## 2.3. The Ideal Age of the Animals Used in STZ DM Models

The models used for T1DM and T2DM are both for rats than for mices 7-10 weeks [44, 52]. However, most studies have shown that younger animals have less resistance to STZ and respond more intensely to its effects [38].

Rodent DM models have been even using neonatal animals, where the development of hyperglycemia, glucose intolerance, and insulin deficiency is an insidious process. These animals are initially almost asymptomatic, with DM only manifesting itself clearly in early adulthood, during the seventh to eighth week of age, coinciding with puberty [53]. All the major studies that evaluated this model have produced similar results [54-59]. This occurs because STZ administered in neonatal life causes regeneration, however, there is a partial loss of β-cell mass and function [60]. These findings suggest that STZ administered to neonatal animals can be used to induce experimental DM and also as a model for studies of β-cell neogenesis and/or proliferation [61]. However, the pathophysiological mechanism involved in this regeneration is unclear [60]. It has also been claimed that features of this model may resemble the natural course of type 1 DM (T1DM) in humans [62], since several metabolic defects and a functional impairment of adipose tissue are present [62], producing "permanent" disruption of carbohydrate metabolism and aggravation of diabetic status [53].

One of the disadvantages of the method is the high mortality (30–50%) found in some studies administering 100 mg/kg STZ on the day of birth [63].

On the other hand, the administration of 70 mg/kg of STZ intraperitoneally to rats on day 4 of their postnatal life has been employed in some studies [57-59] and did not result in high mortality rates [57].

## 2.4. The Sex of Animals Used in STZ DM Models

In humans, the prevalence of DM is higher males than females [64]. This is because female sex steroids protect β-cells from injury [65, 66]. This is also the case in rodent models, as both sexes of mice have been shown to develop a vulnerability to STZ-induced insulin deficiency when estradiol production was suppressed [65]. For this reason, most studies use male animals [10, 11, 43, 49, 65].

### 2.5. The Nutritional Status of Animals Prior to STZ Administration

There are 2 main protocols used to generate rodent STZ models of DM whereby the rats are fed *ad libitum* throughout the experiment [68, 69], or they are fasted for 4–6 h before injection of STZ [45].

The problem with fasting for several days (protocols that recommend multiple doses of STZ) is the generation of metabolic stress [68].

Moreover, differences in insulin concentration have been identified when caloric restriction was used more frequently [70, 71]. This was demonstrated in a study showing that intermittent daily fasting for 15 h over a period of 30 days opposed the development of glucose intolerance or frank DM. This may have been due to the weight and adiposity reduction that occurred in this model [72, 73].

However, the administration of a single STZ dose to fasted animals can be advantageous because fasting minimizes competition between STZ and glucose for low affinity GLUT2 transporters on β-cells [74]. Thus, several researchers recommend overnight fasting before administration of STZ [45-48, 50].

Taken together, the above findings indicate that study protocols employing multiple doses of STZ should use non-fasted animals, since nutritional status does not seem to affect the results [68]. However, for protocols using single doses of STZ, the animals should be fasted for 4–6 h [45-48, 50].

### 2.6. Preparation of STZ Before Administration

STZ needs to be diluted in buffer solution before it can be used to induce DM. There is a consensus that filtered 0.1 M citrate buffer, pH 4.5, should be used [75]. Moreover, the typical recommendation is to avoid exposure of the STZ to light, and to administer it within 10 min of dissolution, due to its instability in solution [48, 50, 76, 77].

## Unit 3 - Dosage and Associations

### 3.1. Single Dose of STZ

STZ is capable of producing mild to severe types of DM, depending on the dosage used. A single dose of STZ is commonly used to induce T1DM, although this has also been used to induce T2DM [78, 79]. These models are generally used to screen new anti-diabetic molecules [80] and to investigate diabetes-related cardiomyopathy [81]. The disadvantage of the method is the instability of the resulting diabetic condition. Moreover, sudden death is caused in approximately 10–20% of the animals treated due to the elevated blood glucose and STZ toxicity [82].

The recommended dose varies between different rodent species. Generally, the dose is between 50 and 85 mg/kg in Wistar or Sprague-Dawley rats [42, 83–86]. In mice, the dose can vary between 130 and 225 mg/kg [78, 87]. A study involving different strains of mice showed that approximately 100 mg/kg was ideal for the induction of T2DM, whilst 200 mg/kg induced T1DM [78]. However, the administration of multiple low STZ doses in conjunction with a high-fat diet is currently the preferred method to induce T2DM in rodent models.

Since most of the studies evaluated in this review have shown that higher STZ doses were required to induce T1DM, we suggest the use of 200 mg/kg intraperitoneally for mice [78, 87] and 65 mg/kg intraperitoneally for rats, which is the dose commonly used [42, 84–86].

### 3.2. Multiple Low Doses of STZ

Multiple doses of STZ have been widely used, especially in T2DM models [79], although this approach may also be used to generate T1DM [88]. The main advantages of this method are the progressive destruction of pancreatic β-cells, and the decreased animal morbidity and mortality, compared with a single dose of STZ [78]. The main protocols that use multiple low doses of STZ also use diets high in fat, fructose or nicotinamide. Details of these techniques are described below.

### 3.3. High-Fat Diet and STZ

As the prevalence of T2DM is rising worldwide due to increased obesity levels [89], animal models capable of matching the main characteristics of this disease are required. The use of low doses of STZ in animals on a high-fat diet has been increasingly seen in rodent models, because STZ treatment alone did not decrease hepatic insulin sensitivity sufficiently [90].

This approach was first reported in the 1970s [91] and has many advantages as an animal model of T2DM that represents the natural history and metabolic characteristics of the human syndrome more closely and responds to pharmaceutical treatment [92].

In general, this model exacerbates mild STZ-induced DM, primarily by increasing hyperglycemia [90, 91] and hepatic lipid deposition [67, 91].

The mechanism of action involves hepatic insulin resistance in the presence of mild insulin deficiency [93, 94]. Moreover, an alteration in cell membrane composition induced by the high-fat diet may also contribute to decreased insulin-stimulated glucose clearance [95]. Such membrane changes may also be important in regulating T cell-mediated immunity in insulin-dependent DM [96].

There is currently extensive divergence in research protocols involving high-fat diets, especially with respect to the period of administration, the type of diet, and STZ dosage. An investigation of the effects of animal age, STZ dosage, and the high-fat diet administration period was reported in 1993 [38]. The authors compared administration of 0, 30, 60, and 90 mg/kg STZ on the day of birth, followed by a high-fat diet, and concluded that low-dose STZ and a high-fat diet for at least 3 weeks were ideal conditions for a T2DM model. Rats exposed to STZ at 3 months of age showed higher hyperglycemia than rats treated at 6 months of age, indicating that older rats were more resistant to development of T2DM using this approach. The authors speculated that very low dose neonatal STZ administration impaired glucose tolerance through decreased overall insulin responses. This may be due to a reduction in β-cell number, rather than an alteration in the activity of these cells [38]. After this study, several other protocols were suggested in the literature, all of which reported successful generation of DM models [44, 92, 97-100]. Before detailing the major protocols, we will describe the main types of high-fat diets employed in these studies.

### 3.4. High-Fat Diets

The amount of fat in the diet has been varied from 30% to 70% using a range of protocols [44, 92, 97-100]. Laboratory animal diets have been classified into three major categories: chows (cereal-based diet), semi-purified, and chemically defined diets. These may exert significant independent effects on the phenotypes measured in any research protocol [101]. The most suitable diet category for this type of experiment is semi-purified, because this is formulated from refined nutrient ingredients, can be intentionally modified to meet the researcher's needs, contains negligible extraneous material, and shows very little batch-to-batch variation [102].

A recent study compared a range of metabolic parameters in male Wistar rats administered different diets for a period of 12 weeks [102]. This study indicated that diets containing more than 50% fat were not ideal for some types of research studies, for example those studying the effects of a drug, nutraceutical, or gene mutation on obesity, because it might be more difficult to prevent or reverse the effects of a very high-fat diet. The authors concluded that the ideal high-fat diet should contain 45% kcal fat at most, provided by 37.5 g soya oil and 200 g lard/kg diet. This produced appropriate metabolic alterations for research studies on diet-induced metabolic disorders using Wistar rats [102].

There is no published research investigating the ideal time that the rats should remain on a high-fat diet before or after administration of STZ. Protocols vary, with an average of 2–8 weeks of high-fat diet [44, 92, 97-100]. There is evidence that the response of young rats to STZ is more similar to that of diabetic humans, with insulin resistance and increased hyperglycemia.

Thus, if insulin resistance occurs within an average time of 2–4 weeks, it would be better to administer STZ at this stage, before the animals age further, decreasing the probability of successful generation of a DM model [38, 103].

### 3.5. The Optimal Dosage of STZ with a High-Fat Diet

The literature describes the usage of a broad range of STZ doses, as well as different routes of administration. Both the intraperitoneal and intravenous routes have been used in several studies [44, 92, 97-100]. The greatest advantage of intraperitoneal administration is the ease of administration. In contrast to intravenous administration, it does not require general anesthesia. On the other hand, intravenous administration results in more rapid and greater drug absorption [104]. However, there will be losses reported in the literature on the use of the intraperitoneal route.

Reported doses of STZ administered in association with a high-fat diet range between 15 and 40 mg/kg [44, 92, 97-100]. Both single dose [43, 93] and multi-dose, low concentration, regimens have been reported [90, 95].

The first study employing multiple STZ dosing in this type of model was described in 1978 [105]. This study reported increased serum glucose levels using this methodology [105]. It was subsequently reported that this model activated a detectable immune response during STZ dosing which, although low, may be pathologically meaningful as it is also observed in humans [106]. Furthermore, insulin resistance was also observed in this model [106].

The main advantages of models employing multiple low-dose STZ are: i) the induction of a combination of toxicity and immune response, with progressive hyperglycemia [107]; ii) the involvement of immunological adjuvants, playing a synergistic role in prompting the induction of DM with multiple low doses of STZ, analogous to the decompensated phase of human T2DM [108]. For these reasons, many protocols have proposed the use of high-fat diet associated with multiple low-doses of STZ to achieve an optimal model of T2DM [107-111]. The average dose for this protocol generally ranges between 20 and 30 mg/kg [92, 107, 110], for 2 to 5 days [92, 107, 108, 110].

Although the use of multiple doses of STZ appears to be most advantageous for generation of T2DM models, a single dose of STZ associated with high-fat diet may also produce models similar to T2DM [44, 97, 98]. One of the advantages of this method is the reduced numbers of operative sessions with the animal. The average recommended doses for this method are 30–40 mg/kg [44, 97, 98]. An important aspect to consider is that the higher the STZ dose administered, the greater and faster the destruction of pancreatic β-cells. As rapid β-cell destruction is not ideal for models of T2DM, the lowest possible dose should be employed [107].

Possibly due to methodological differences, some studies did not find that high-fat diet associated with STZ led to insulin resistance [47, 112]. In 1983, the effects of high beef tallow, high corn oil, or low-fat diets were compared in normal and STZ-induced diabetic adult male breeder rats. The rats were fed with the test diets *ad libitum* for 2 months, but no effects on plasma glucose or insulin levels were observed. One potential reason for this was that the high-fat diet contained only 21% corn oil. Most studies have employed fat contents of 30–60% [94, 95, 113].

Another recent study showed that with a 60% fat diet with 25 mg/kg STZ, plasma insulin concentrations were not significantly different to control animals. However, when the STZ dose was increased to 30 mg/kg and administered with a 60% fat diet, the mice developed high levels of glucose and insulin resistance [47].

From the results of these studies, it can be concluded that to achieve an ideal model of T2DM with hyperglycemia and insulin resistance, the optimal protocol would include: 1) treatment of the animals with a high-fat diet containing 30–50% fat for 2 to 4 weeks [38, 102, 103]; 2) administration of multiple doses of STZ intraperitoneally at a dose of approximately 25 mg/kg for 2–5 consecutive days [92, 107, 108]. The use of pilot studies for each type of research is also necessary in order to identify the best supplier, and the best strain and weight of the animals.

### 3.6. The Combination of Fructose with STZ

Although the use of high-fat diets can produce successful models of T2DM, this type of specially-formulated diet can be difficult for many researchers to access due to a lack of food ingredient availability or a lack of facilities to feed specially formulated diets. Thus, the addition of fructose provides a good alternative to the high-fat diet, especially in countries where research funds and resources are limited [42].

Exposure of liver to large quantities of fructose and fats leads to rapid stimulation of lipogenesis, resulting in triglyceride accumulation, reduced insulin sensitivity, and hepatic insulin resistance/glucose intolerance [114]. Protocols involving the administration of fructose with low doses of STZ have not been widely used.

The use of 35 mg/kg STZ associated with a high-fat diet, plus fructose solution (20%) for 6 weeks has been investigated [67]. The authors concluded that this model was interesting because it mimicked human T2DM. However, this model is not practical and does not solve the problem of possible difficulties for researchers with limited access to standardized high-fat diets [67].

Another recently suggested protocol showed that a single low dose of STZ associated with fructose administration produced favorable results for a T2DM model. The authors suggested the use of 40 mg/kg STZ with a 10% fructose solution for 2 weeks. This model was advantageous because of its rapid and successful induction of T2DM and partial pancreatic β-cell dysfunction. Moreover, the model produced a stable diabetic condition over an 11-week experimental period and could therefore be used for both acute and chronic research studies, as well as routine pharmacological screening of anti-T2DM therapies. It is also easy to develop and highly cost-effective [42].

Although this method appears to be interesting, it is not yet possible to ensure its reliability due to the small number of published studies.

### 3.7. The Combination of Nicotinamide with STZ

Nicotinamide can be used in combination with STZ to induce DM. This approach was first proposed in 1998 and its mechanism of action involves nicotinamide partially protecting against the β-cytotoxic effect of STZ [115].

One published protocol utilized 2 doses of 100 mg/kg STZ intraperitoneally, followed by nicotinamide (240 mg/kg), and associated with a high fat diet [51]. The researchers argued that combined administration of STZ and nicotinamide caused partial depletion of pancreatic insulin, whilst the high-fat diet led to insulin resistance in this model [51]. However, the method is technically demanding, since the animals were injected with 2 drugs, in addition to requiring a high-fat diet. In addition, some studies have shown that the combination of STZ and nicotinamide induced mutagenic and carcinogenic effects in rats [35, 37].

## UNIT 4 – DM MODELS IN PREGNANT RATS

For some types of research, models of DM using pregnant rats are required. These studies are needed to evaluate the hormonal and metabolic changes that occur during pregnancy. Although using animal models is associated with certain limitations, this type of research is not feasible in humans for ethical reasons [59]. A report dealing with reference data on placental development in rats [116] showed that a combined data set on placental morphology and maternal blood parameters provided a powerful tool for the recognition of abnormal pregnancies [116]. This type of approach may therefore be of interest in producing a standardized animal model to mimic the conditions of diabetes in human pregnancy as closely as possible.

DM during pregnancy may be divided into clinical DM and gestational DM [117]. Wistar or Sprague-Dawley strains are usually used to model hyperglycemia in pregnant rats. Human T2DM and gestational DM are reproduced in animals by administration of different doses of STZ in the neonatal period [118, 119], before mating [120], or during pregnancy [121, 122].

This model has peculiar characteristics. The genotoxicity of STZ was studied in pregnant rats where one group received 100 mg/kg STZ intraperitoneally to produce mild diabetes, and the other group received 40 mg/kg intravenously to produce severe diabetes. This study showed more evident genotoxicity in rats receiving 40 mg/kg STZ intravenously [123].

In addition, fetuses from diabetic rat mothers show growth retardation and their chondrocytes showed reduced responsiveness to various growth factors, as compared to cells from normal fetuses [122]. On the other hand, this model is also reported to produce an elevated long-term risk for macrosomia, which is also found in humans [124].

## 4.2. Ideal STZ Dosage for Induction of DM in Pregnant Rats

Like other protocols discussed in this review, a variety of STZ doses have been utilized in pregnant rats. There is no consensus regarding the optimal STZ dose, the number of doses, or administration route.

The recommended dose of STZ varies primarily depending on the model. The administration of 70 mg/kg of STZ intraperitoneally to rats on day 4 of postnatal life has been reported in some studies [57-59] and this did not seem to cause a high mortality rate [57]. However, this model is not very reliable, because there is evidence of pancreatic cell regeneration after STZ injection, and the pathophysiological mechanism involved in this regeneration is unclear [60].

For administration before mating, the same doses recommended for normal rats can be used, as described previously. However, there was a report that the utilization of 100mg/kg STZ intravenously in combination with high diet fat is recommended in this case [76].

The best model for studies of DM in pregnancy appears to be generated by injection of STZ on the first days of gestation, because there is a reduction in insulin levels during the pregnancy. Furthermore, most fetuses showed macrosomia and high serum levels of glucose and insulin on the first day of life. These findings suggested that this model was the most successful at reproducing human pathogenesis [60].

Multiple low doses of STZ would be contraindicated in this model because of their high variability in glucose levels, the normal insulin response to a glucose load, the absence of fetal macrosomia, and the inconsistent effect on fetal insulin concentrations [116]. The optimal STZ dose reported was 30 mg/kg, administered either intraperitoneally [121] or intravenously [124]. For this protocol (in rats on the first days of gestation), there are no studies clear analyzing the advantages or disadvantages of fasting, or high-fat diets. However, most researchers seem to provide food and water ad libitum and do not use high-fat diets [124, 125].

## Unit 5 – Final Considerations

From this review, it can be concluded that although there are many different protocols described in the literature, it has been difficult to standardize the method, producing an ideal model. In addition, there is a gap in the literature regarding the genotoxicity of STZ in more recently developed protocols, particularly those involving a high-fat diet.

It is clear that the researcher must select the most appropriate protocol for the type of research proposed and the available resources. However, there are some important considerations for all experimental rodent models of STZ-induced DM:

1 Whilst there is no agreement on the best animal strain for STZ-induced DM models, it is important to consider which animal supplier is used, because each vendor provides a unique subline [49]. Pilot studies are therefore useful to identify the optimal supplier.
2 Younger animals should ideally be chosen, since they respond more intensely to STZ [38].
3 Unless the study is related to female sex hormones, male animals should be used for the majority of studies [10, 11, 44, 50, 67].
4 The recommended STZ dilution buffer is sterile-filtered 0.1 M citrate buffer, pH 4.5. Moreover, this solution should be kept in the dark and administered within 10 min of dissolution [75].

We also conclude, based on the research reviewed here, that one of the best protocols for a model of T1DM would involve overnight fasting for 4–6 h [45] followed by administration of 200 mg/kg STZ intraperitoneally for mice [78, 87], or 65 mg/kg intraperitoneally for rats [42, 84–86]. This method is the simplest and has shown good results in the studies reviewed. However, the combination of a high-fat diet with this model is also interesting when possible.

For models of T2DM, the best protocol appeared to involve a high-fat (30–50%) diet [102] for 2–4 weeks [38, 103], and multiple doses of STZ (25 mg/kg) administered intraperitoneally [107] on 2–5 consecutive days [92].

Finally, although there are no well-established protocols for gestational DM models, it appeared best to administer 30 mg/kg STZ either intravenously or intraperitoneally on the first days of gestation [121, 124, 125]. However, more studies need to be conducted to optimize this model.

## Acknowledgments

We acknowledge PROPe (0323/019/13-PROPe/CDC) and Fapesp (2012/02083-8) by provided technical assistance.

## REFERENCES

[1] Vavra, J. J., Deboer, C., Dietz, A., Hanka, L. J., Sokolski, W. T. Streptozotocin, a new antibacterial antibiotic. *Antibiot. Annu.* 1959;7:230–5.

[2] Herr, R. R., Jahnke, A. D., Argoudelis, A. D. The structure of Streptozotocin. *J. Am. Chem. Soc.* 1967;89:4808–9.

[3] Hardegger, E., Meier, A., Stoos, A. A preparative synthesis of Streptozotocin. *Helv. Chim. Acta.* 1969;52:2555–60.

[4] Hessler, E. J., Jahnke, H. K. Improved synthesis of streptozotocin. *J. Org. Chem.* 1970; 35: 245-6.

[5] Murray-Lyon, I. M., Eddleston, A. L., Williams, R., Brown, M., Hogbin, B. M., Bennett, A., Edwards, J. C., Taylor, K. W. Treatment of multiple-hormone-producing malignant islet-cell tumour with streptozotocin. *Lancet.* 1968;26:895-8.

[6] Arnould, Y., Ooms, H. A., Bastenie, P. A. Treatment of insulinoma with streptozotocin. *Lancet.* 1969;7607:1210-1.

[7] Schreibman, P. H., De Koliren, L. G., Arky, R. A. Metastatic insulinoma treated with streptozotocin. *Annals Internal Med.* 1971;74:399-403.

[8] Bolzán, A. D., Bianchi, M. S. Genotoxicity of streptozotocin. *Mutat. Res.* 2002; 512: 121-34.

[9] Rossini, A. A., Like, A. A., Chick, W. L., Appel, M. C., Cahill, Jr G. F. Studies of streptozotocin-induced insulitis and diabetes. *Proceed. Nat. Acad. Sci. US.* 1977; 74: 2485–9.

[10] Cintra, L. T., da Silva Facundo, A. C., Azuma, M. M., Sumida, D. H., Astolphi, R. D., Bomfim, S. R., Narciso, L. G., Gomes-Filho, J. E. Pulpal and periodontal diseases increase triglyceride levels in diabetic rats. *Clin. Oral Investig.* 2013;17:1595-9.

[11] Cintra, L. T., Samuel, R. O., Facundo, A. C., Prieto, A. K., Sumida, D. H., Bomfim, S. R., Souza, J. C., Dezan-Júnior, E., Gomes-Filho, J. E. Relationships between oral infections and blood glucose concentrations or HbA1c levels in normal and diabetic rats. *Int. Endod. J.* 2013; doi: 10.1111/iej.12136. [Epub. ahead of print].

[12] Kesavan, S. K., Bhat, S., Golegaonkar, S. B., Jagadeeshaprasad, M. G., Deshmukh, A. B., Patil, H. S., Bhosale, S. D., Shaikh, M. L., Thulasiram, H. V., Boppana, R., Kulkarni, M. J. Proteome wide reduction in AGE modification in streptozotocin induced diabetic mice by hydralazine mediated transglycation. *Sci. Rep.* 2013;15:2941.

[13] Bennett, R. A., Pegg, A. E. Alkylation of DNA in rat tissues following administration of streptozotocin. *Cancer Res.* 1981;41:2786-90.

[14] Chang, A. Y., Schneider, D. I. Hepatic enzyme activities in streptozotocin-diabetic rats before and after insulin treatment. *Diabetes.* 1971;20:71-7.

[15] Dean, P. M., Matthews, E. K. Electrical activity in pancreatic islet cells: effect of ions. *J. Physiol.* 1970;210:265-75.

[16] Dean, P. M., Matthews, E. K. The biophysical properties of pancreatic islet cells; effect of diabetogenic agents. *Diabetologia.* 1972;8:173-8.

[17] Kawada, J. New hypotheses for the mechanisms of streptozotocin and alloxan inducing diabetes mellitus. *Yakugaku Zasshi.* 1992;112:773-91.

[18] Ghaffari, T., Nouri, M., Saei, A. A., Rashidi, M. R. Aldehyde and Xanthine Oxidase Activities in Tissues of Streptozotocin-Induced Diabetic Rats: Effects of Vitamin E and Selenium Supplementation. *Biol. Traço Elem. Res*. 2012;147:217-25.

[19] Kröncke, K. D., Fehsel, K., Sommer, A., Rodriguez, M. L., Kolb-Bachofen, V. Nitric oxide generation during cellular metabolization of the diabetogenic N-methyl-N-nitroso-urea streptozotozin contributes to islet cell DNA damage. *Biol. Chem. Hoppe. Seyler*. 1995;376:179-85.

[20] Morgan, N. G., Cable, H. C., Newcombe, N. R., Williams, G. T. Treatment of cultured pancreatic B-cells with streptozotocin induces cell death by apoptosis. *Bioscience Reports*. 1994;14:243-50.

[21] Flodström, M., Tyrberg, B., Eizirik, D. L., Sandler, S. Reduced sensitivity of inducible nitric oxide synthase-deficient mice to multiple low-dose streptozotocin-induced diabetes. *Diabetes*. 1999;48:706-13.

[22] González, E., Roselló-Catafau, J., Jawerbaum, A., Sinner, D., Pustovrh, C., Vela, J., White, V., Xaus, C., Peralta, C., Gimeno, M. Pancreatic nitric oxide and oxygen free radicals in the early stages of streptozotocin-induced diabetes mellitus in the rat. *Braz. J. Med. Biol. Res*. 2000;33:1335-42.

[23] Gandy, S. E., Buse, M. G., Crouch, R. K. Protective role of superoxide dismutase against diabetogenic drugs. *J. Clin. Invest*. 1982;70(3):650-8.

[24] Arison, R. N., Feudale, E. L. Induction of renal tumour by Streptozotocin in rats. *Nature*. 1967;214:1254–5.

[25] Sugimura, T., Fujimura, S. Tumour production in glandular stomach of rat by N-methyl-N'-nitro-N-nitrosoguanidine. *Nature*. 1967;216:943-4.

[26] Kolbye, S. M., Legator, M. S. Mutagenic activity of streptozotocin. *Mutat. Res*. 1968;6: 387-9.

[27] Gabridge, M. G., Denunzio, A., Legator, M. S. Microbial mutagenicity of streptozotocin in animal-mediated assays. *Nature*. 1969;22:68-70.

[28] Mossman, B. T., Wilson, G. L., Craighead, J. E. Chlorozocin. A diabetogenic analogue of streptozocin with dissimilar mechanisms of action on pancreatic beta cells. *Diabetes*. 1985; 34:602-10.

[29] Ohkuwa, T., Sato, Y., Naoi, M. Hydroxyl radical formation in diabetic rats induced by streptozotocin. *Life Sci*. 1995;56:1789-98. Erratum in: *Life Sci*. 1995;57:1325.

[30] Drabløs, F., Feyzi, E., Aas, P. A., Vaagbø, C. B., Kavli, B., Bratlie, M. S., Peña-Diaz, J., Otterlei, M., Slupphaug, G., Krokan, H. E. Alkylation damage in DNA and RNA--repair mechanisms and medical significance. *DNA Repair* (Amst.). 2004;3:1389-407.

[31] Tjälve, H., Löfberg, B. Extrahepatic sites of metabolism of carbon tetrachloride in rats. *Chem. Biol. Interact*. 1983;46:299-316.

[32] Erickson, L. C., Bradley, M. O., Kohn, K. W. Measurements of DNA damage in Chinese hamster cells treated with equitoxic and equimutagenic doses of nitrosoureas. *Cancer Res*. 1978;38:3379–84.

[33] Yamamoto, H., Uchigata, Y., Okamoto, H. Streptozotocin and alloxan induce DNA strand breaks and poly (ADP-ribose) synthetase in pancreatic islets. *Nature*. 1981;294: 284-6.

[34] Rakieten, N., Gordon, B. S., Cooney, D. A., Davis, R. D., Schein, P. S. Renal tumorigenic action of Streptozotocin in rats. *Cancer Chemother. Rep*. 1968;52:563–7.

[35] Rakieten, N., Gordon, B. S., Beaty, A., Cooney, D. A., Davis, R. D., Schein, P. S. Pancreatic islet cell tumors produced by the combined action of Streptozotocin and nicotinamide. *Proc. Soc. Exp. Biol. Med.* 1971;137:280–3.

[36] Iwase, M., Nunoi, K., Sadoshima, S., Kikuchi, M., Fujishima, M. Liver, kidney and is let cell tumors in spontaneously hypertensive and normotensive rats treated with Streptozotocin. *Tohoku J. Exp. Med.* 1989;159:83–90.

[37] Rakieten, N., Gordon, B. S., Beaty, A., Cooney, D. A., Schein, P. S. Modification of renal tumorigenic effect of Streptozotocin by nicotinarnide: spontaneous reversibiJity of Streptozotocin diabetes. *Proc. Soc. Exp. Biol. Med.* 1976;151:356–61.

[38] Wiersma, M. M., Bakker, I. M., Radder, J. K. Effect of high fat feeding on glucose tolerance in neonatally streptozotocin-treated rats at 3 and 6 months of age. *Ann. NY Acad. Sci.* 1993;683:228-36.

[39] Vikram, A., Tripathi, D. N., Ramarao, P., Jena, G. B. Evaluation of streptozotocin genotoxicity in rats from different ages using the micronucleus assay. *Regul. Toxicol. Pharmaco.* 2007;49:238-44.

[40] Kraynak, A. R., Storer, R. D., Jensen, R. D., Kloss, M. W., Soper, K. A., Clair, J. H., DeLuca, J. G., Nichols, W. W., Eydelloth, R. S. Extent and persistence of streptozotocin-induced DNA damage and cell proliferation in rat kidney as determined by in vivo alkaline elution and BrdUrd labeling assays. *Toxicol. Appl. Pharmacol.* 1995; 135:279-86.

[41] Grodsky, G. M., Anderson, C. E., Coleman, D. L., Craighead, J. E., Gerritsen, G. C., Hansen, C. T., Herberg, L., Howard, C. F. Jr, Lernmark, A., Matschinsky, F. M., Rayfield, E., Riley, W. J., Rossini, A. A. Metabolic and underlying causes of diabetes mellitus. *Diabetes.* 1982;31:45-53.

[42] Islam, M. S., Wilson, R. D. Experimentally induced rodent models of type 2 diabetes. *Methods Mol. Biol.* 2012;933:161-74.

[43] Tesch, G. H., Allen, T. J. Rodent models of streptozotocin-induced diabetic nephropathy. *Nephrology* (Carlton). 2007;12:261-6.

[44] Reed, M. J., Meszaros, K., Entes, L. J., Claypool, M. D., Pinkett, J. G., Gadbois, T. M., Reaven, G. M. A new rat model of type 2 diabetes: the fat-fed, streptozotocin-treated rat. *Metabolism.* 2000;49:1390-4.

[45] Morrow, T. J. Animal models of painful diabetic neuropathy: the STZ rat model. *Curr. Protoc. Neurosci.* 2004; Chapter 9:Unit 9.18.

[46] Salama, R. M., Schaalan, M. F., Elkoussi, A. A., Khalifa, A. E. Potential Utility of Sodium Selenate as an Adjunct to Metformin in Treating Type II Diabetes Mellitus in Rats: A Perspective on Protein Tyrosine Phosphatase. *Biomed. Res. Int.* 2013;2013: 231378.

[47] Mansor, L. S., Gonzalez, E. R., Cole, M. A., Tyler, D. J., Beeson, J. H., Clarke, K., Carr, C. A., Heather, L. C. Cardiac metabolism in a new rat model of type 2 diabetes using high-fat diet with low dose streptozotocin. *Cardiovasc. Diabetol.* 2013;24:136.

[48] Ferhatovic, L., Banozic, A., Kostic, S., Kurir, T. T., Novak, A., Vrdoljak, L., Heffer, M., Sapunar, D., Puljak, L. Expression of calcium/calmodulin-dependent protein kinase II and pain-related behavior in rat models of type 1 and type 2 diabetes. *Anesth. Analg.* 2013;116:712-21.

[49] Graham, M. L., Janecek, J. L., Kittredge, J. A., Hering, B. J., Schuurman, H. J. The streptozotocin-induced diabetic nude mouse model: differences between animals from different sources. *Comp. Med.* 2011;61:356-60.

[50] Okamoto, T., Kanemoto, N., Ohbuchi, Y., Okano, M., Fukui, H., Sudo, T. Characterization of STZ-Induced Type 2 Diabetes in Zucker Fatty Rats. *Exp. Anim.* 2008; 57:335-45.

[51] Nakamura, T., Terajima, T., Ogata, T., Ueno, K., Hashimoto, N., Ono, K., Yano, S. Establishment and pathophysiological characterization of type 2 diabetic mouse model produced by streptozotocin and nicotinamide. *Biol. Pharm. Bull.* 2006;29:1167-74.

[52] Novikova, L., Smirnova, I. V., Rawal, S., Dotson, A. L., Benedict, S. H., Stehno-Bittel, L. Variations in rodent models of type 1 diabetes: islet morphology. *J. Diabetes Res.* 2013;2013:965832.

[53] Takada, J., Machado, M. A., Peres, S. B., Brito, L. C., Borges-Silva, C. N., Costa, C. E., Fonseca-Alaniz, M. H., Andreotti, S., Lima, F. B. Neonatal streptozotocin-induced diabetes mellitus: a model of insulin resistance associated with loss of adipose mass. *Metabolism.* 2007;56:977-84.

[54] Bonner-Weir, S., Trent, D. F., Honey, R. N., Weir, G. C. Responses of neonatal rat islets to streptozotocin. Limited B-cell regeneration and hyperglycemia. *Diabetes.* 1981; 30:64–69.

[55] Tsuji, K., Taminato, T., Usami, M., Ishida, H., N. Kitano, Fukumoto, H., Koh, L., Kurose, T., Yamada, Y., Yano, H. Characteristic features of insulin secretion in the streptozotocin-induced NIDDM rat model. *Metabolism.* 1988;37:1040–4.

[56] Wang, R. N., Bouwens, L., Klöppel, G. Beta-cell proliferation in normal and streptozotocin-treated newborn rats: site, dynamics and capacity. *Diabetologia.* 1994; 37:1088–96.

[57] Thyssen, S., Arany, E., Hill, D. J. Ontogeny of regeneration of β-cells in the neonatal rat after treatment with streptozotocin. *Endocrinology.*2006;147:2346–56.

[58] Nicholson, J. M., Arany, E. J., Hill, D. J. Changes in islet microvasculature following streptozotocin-induced β-cell loss and subsequent replacement in the neonatal rat. *Experim. Biol. Med.* 2010;235:189–98.

[59] Liang, X. D., Guo, Y. Y., Sun, M., Ding, Y., Wang, N., Yuan, L., De, W. Streptozotocin-induced expression of Ngn3 and Pax4 in neonatal rat pancreatic α-cells. *World. J. Gastroen.* 2011;17:2812–20.

[60] Damasceno, D. C., Sinzato, Y. K., Bueno, A., Netto, A. O., Dallaqua, B., Gallego, F. Q., Iessi, I. L., Corvino, S. B., Serrano, R. G., Marini, G., Piculo, F., Calderon, I. M., Rudge, M. V. Mild diabetes models and their maternal-fetal repercussions. *J. Diabetes Res.* 2013;2013:473575.

[61] Portha, B., Blondel, O., Serradas, P., McEvoy, R., Giroix, M. H., Kergoat, M., Bailbe, D. The rat models of non-insulin dependent diabetes induced by neonatal streptozotocin. *Diabete Metab.* 1989;15:61-75.

[62] De Oliveira, A. C., Andreotti, S., Farias Tda, S., Torres-Leal, F. L., de Proença, A. R., Campaña, A. B., de Souza, A. H., Sertié, R. A., Carpinelli, A. R., Cipolla-Neto, J., Lima, F. B. Metabolic disorders and adipose tissue insulin responsiveness in neonatally STZ-induced diabetic rats are improved by long-term melatonin treatment. *Endocrinology.* 2012;153:2178-88.

[63] Portha, B., Levacher, C., Picon, L., Rosselin, G. Diabetogenic effect of streptozotocin in the rat during the perinatal period. *Diabetes*. 1974;23:889-95.

[64] Wild, S., Roglic, G., Green, A., Sicree, R., King, H. (2004) Global prevalence of diabetes: estimates for the year 2000 and projections for 2030. *Diabetes Care*. 27:1047–53.

[65] Le May, C., Chu, K., Hu, M., Ortega, C. S., Simpson, E. R., Korach, K. S., Tsai, M. J., Mauvais-Jarvis, F. Estrogens protect pancreatic beta-cells from apoptosis and prevent insulin-deficient diabetes mellitus in mice. *Proc. Natl. Acad. Sci. US*. 2006;103:9232-7.

[66] Liu, S., Kilic, G., Meyers, M. S., Navarro, G., Wang, Y., Oberholzer, J., Mauvais-Jarvis, F. Oestrogens improve human pancreatic islet transplantation in a mouse model of insulin deficient diabetes. *Diabetologia*. 2013;56:370-81.

[67] Schaalan, M., El-Abhar, H. S., Barakat, M., El-Denshary, E. S. Westernized-like-diet-fed rats: effect on glucose homeostasis, lipid profile, and adipocyte hormones and their modulation by rosiglitazone and glimepiride. *J. Diabetes Comp*. 2009;23:199-208.

[68] Chaudhry, Z. Z., Morris, D. L., Moss, D. R., Sims, E. K., Chiong, Y., Kono, T., Evans-Molina, C. Streptozotocin is equally diabetogenic whether administered to fed or fasted mice. *Lab. Anim*. 2013;47:257-65.

[69] Chia, J. S., McRae, J. L., Thomas, H. E., Fynch, S., Elkerbout, L., P. Colina, Murray-Segal, L., Robson, S. C., Chen, J. F., d'Apice, A. J., Cowan, P. J., Dwyer, K. M. The protective effects of CD39 overexpression in multiple low-dose streptozotocin-induced diabetes in mice. *Diabetes*. 2013;62:2026-35.

[70] Dean, D. J., Gazdag, A. C., Wetter, T. J., Cartee, G. D. Comparison of the effects of 20 days and 15 months of calorie restriction on male Fischer 344 rats. *Aging Clin. Exp. Res*. 1998;10:303–7.

[71] Wetter, T. J., Gazdag, A. C., Dean, D. J., Cartee, G. D. Effect of calorie restriction on in vivo glucose metabolism by individual tissues in rats. *Am. J. Physiol*. 1999; 276:E728-38.

[72] Belkacemi, L., Selselet-Attou, G., Louchami, K., Sener, A., Malaisse, W. J. Intermittent fasting modulation of the diabetic syndrome in sand rats. II. In vivo investigations. *Int. J. Mol. Med*. 2010;26:759-65.

[73] Belkacemi, L., Selselet-Attou, G., Hupkens, E., Nguidjoe, E., Louchami, K., Sener, A., Malaisse, W. J. Intermittent fasting modulation of the diabetic syndrome in streptozotocin-injected rats. *Int. J. Endocrinol*. 2012;2012:962012.

[74] Marks, J., Carvou, N. J., Debnam, E. S., Srai, S. K., Unwin, R. J. Diabetes increases facilitative glucose uptake and GLUT2 expression at the rat proximal tubule brush border membrane. *J. Physiol*. 2003;553:137-45.

[75] De la Garza-Rodea, A. S., Knaän-Shanzer, S., den Hartigh, J. D., Verhaegen, A. P., van Bekkum, D. W. Anomer-equilibrated streptozotocin solution for the induction of experimental diabetes in mice (Mus musculus). *J. Am. Assoc. Lab. Anim. Sci*. 2010;49: 40-4.

[76] Gutierrez, J. C., Bahamonde, J., Prater, M. R., Yefi, C. P., Holladay, S. D. Production of a type 2 maternal diabetes rodent model using the combination of high-fat diet and moderate dose of streptozocin. *Endocr. Res*. 2010;35:59-70.

[77] Kataoka, M., Kawamuro, Y., Shiraki, N., Miki, R., Sakano, D., Yoshida, T., Yasukawa, T., Kume, K., Kume, S. Recovery from diabetes in neonatal mice after a low-dose streptozotocin treatment. *Biochem. Biophys. Res. Commun*. 2013;430:1103-8.

[78] Hayashi, K., Kojima, R., Ito, M. Strain differences in the diabetogenic activity of streptozotocin in mice. *Biol. Pharm. Bull.* 2006;29:1110-9.

[79] Ventura-Sobrevilla, J., Boone-Villa, V. D., Aguilar, C. N., Román-Ramos, R., Vega-Avila, E., Campos-Sepúlveda, E., Alarcón-Aguilar, F. Effect of varying dose and administration of streptozotocin on blood sugar in male CD1 mice. *Proc. West Pharmacol. Soc.* 2011;54:5-9.

[80] Luippold, G., Klein, T., Mark, M., Grempler, R. Empagliflozin, a novel potent and selective SGLT-2 inhibitor, improves glycaemic control alone and in combination with insulin in streptozotocin-induced diabetic rats, a model of type 1 diabetes mellitus. *Diabetes Obes. Metab.* 2012; 14:601–7.

[81] Bugger, H., Abel, E. D. Rodent models of diabetic cardiomyopathy. *Dis. Model Mech.* 2009; 2:454-66.

[82] Sakata, N., Yoshimatsu, G., Tsuchiya, H., Egawa, S., Unno, M. Animal models of diabetes mellitus for islet transplantation. *Exp. Diabetes Res.* 2012;2012:256707.

[83] Yang, J., Cherian, M. G. Protective effects of metallothionein on streptozotocin-induced diabetes in rats. *Life Sci.* 1994;55:43-51.

[84] Talbot, S., De Brito Gariépy, H., Saint-Denis, J., Couture, R. Activation of kinin B1 receptor evokes hyperthermia through a vagal sensory mechanism in the rat. *J. Neuroinflam.* 2012;13:214.

[85] Tirgan, N., Kulp, G. A., Gupta, P., Boretsky, A., Wiraszka, T. A., Godley, B., Tilton, R. G., Motamedi, M. Nicotine exposure exacerbates development of cataracts in a type 1 diabetic rat model. *Exp. Diabetes Res.* 2012;2012:349320.

[86] Blaes, N., Pécher, C., Mehrenberger, M., Cellier, E., Praddaude, F., Chevalier, J., Tack, I., Couture, R., Girolami, J. P. Bradykinin inhibits high glucose- and growth factor-induced collagen synthesis in mesangial cells through the B2-kinin receptor. *Am. J. Physiol. Renal Physiol.* 2012;303:F293-303.

[87] Yang, B., Li, M., Shi, Z. G., Feng, Q. Z. Bosentan ameliorates the expression of fibrotic related growth factors and collagen-1 in diabetic mice. *Anadolu Kard. Derg.* 2012;12: 621-7.

[88] Castillo, G. M., Nishimoto-Ashfield, A., Banerjee, A. A., Landolfi, J. A., Lyubimov, A. V., Bolotin, E. M. Omeprazole and PGC-Formulated Heparin Binding Epidermal Growth Factor Normalizes Fasting Blood Glucose and Suppresses Insulitis in Multiple Low Dose Streptozotocin Diabetes Model. *Pharm. Res.* 2013;30:2843-54.

[89] Riobó Serván, P. Obesity and diabetes. *Nutr. Hosp.* 2013;28:138-43.

[90] Traianedes, K., Proietto, J., O'Dea, K. A high-fat diet worsens metabolic control in streptozotocin-treated rats by increasing hepatic glucose production. *Metabolism.* 1992; 41:846-50.

[91] Reaven, E. P., Reaven, G. M. Mechanisms for development of diabetic hypertriglyceridemia in streptozotocin-treated rats. Effect of diet and duration of insulin deficiency. *J. Clin. Invest.* 1974;54:1167-78.

[92] Zhang, M., Lv, X. Y., Li, J., Xu, Z. G., Chen, L. The characterization of high-fat diet and multiple low-dose streptozotocin induced type 2 diabetes rat model. *Exp. Diabetes Res.* 2008;2008:704045.

[93] Portha, B., Giroix, M. H., Picon, L. Effect of diet on glucose tolerance and insulin response in chemically diabetic rats. *Metabolism.* 1982;31:1194-9.

[94] Chisholm, K., O'Dea, K. Effect of short-term consumption of a high-fat, low-carbohydrate diet on metabolic control in insulin-deficient diabetic rats. *Metabolism.* 1987;36:237-43.

[95] Bhandaru, R., Srinivasan, S. R., Radhakrisnamurthy, B., Berenson, G. S. Effects of diabetes and high fat-high cholesterol diet on plasma lipid levels and on erythrocyte membrane composition. *Atherosclerosis*. 1982;42:263-72.

[96] Singh, B., Lauzon, J., Venkatraman, J., Thomson, A. B., Rajotte, R. V., Clandinin, M. T. Effect of high/low dietary linoleic acid levels on the function and fatty acid composition of T-lymphocytes of normal and diabetic rats. *Diabetes Res*. 1988;8(3): 129-34.

[97] Srinivasan, K., Viswanad, B., Asrat, L., Kaul, C. L., Ramarao, P. Combination of high-fat diet-fed and low-dose streptozotocin-treated rat: a model for type 2 diabetes and pharmacological screening. *Pharmacol. Res*. 2005;52:313-20.

[98] Islam, M. S., Choi, H. Nongenetic model of type 2 diabetes: a comparative study. *Pharmacology*. 2007;79:243-9.

[99] Gilbert, E. R., Fu, Z., Liu, D. Development of a nongenetic mouse model of type 2 diabetes. *Exp. Diabetes Res*. 2011;2011:416254.

[100] Xiang, X., Wang, Z., Zhu, Y., Bian, L., Yang, Y. Dosage of streptozocin in inducing rat model of type 2 diabetes mellitus. *Wei Sheng Yan Jiu*. 2010;39(2):138-42.

[101] Newberne, P. M., Sotnikov, A. V. Diet: the neglected variable in chemical safety evaluations. *Toxicol. Pathol*. 1996;24:746–56.

[102] Sasidharan, S. R., Joseph, J. A., Anandakumar, S., Venkatesan, V., Ariyattu Madhavan, C. N., Agarwal, A. An experimental approach for selecting appropriate rodent diets for research studies on metabolic disorders. *Biomed. Res. Int*. 2013;2013:752870.

[103] Korou, L. M., Doulamis, I. P., Tzanetakou, I. P., Mikhailidis, D. P., Perrea, D. N. The effect of biological age on the metabolic responsiveness of mice fed a high-fat diet. *Lab. Anim*. 2013;47:241-4.

[104] Smith, R. V., Wilcox, R. E., Soine, W. H., Riffee, W. H., Baldessarini, R. J., Kula, N. S. Plasma levels of apomorphine following intravenous, intraperitoneal and oral administration to mice and rats. *Res. Commun. Chem. Pathol. Pharmacol*. 1979;24(3): 483-99.

[105] Like, A. A., Rossini, A. A. Streptozotocin-induced pancreatic insulitis: new model of diabetes mellitus. *Science*. 1976;4251:415-7.

[106] McEvoy, R. C., Andersson, J., Sandler, S., Hellerström, C. Multiple low-dose streptozotocin-induced diabetes in the mouse. Evidence for stimulation of a cytotoxic cellular immune response against an insulin-producing beta cell line. *J. Clin. Invest*. 1984;74:715–22.

[107] Kim, E., Sohn, S., Lee, M., Jung, J., Kineman, R. D., Park, S. Differential responses of the growth hormone axis in two rat models of streptozotocin-induced insulinopenic diabetes. *J. Endocrin*. 2006;188:263–70.

[108] Wright, J. R., Jr., Lacy, P. E. Synergistic effects of adjuvants, endotoxin, and fasting on induction of diabetes with multiple low doses of streptozocin in rats. *Diabetes*. 1988; 37: 112–18.

[109] Kannan, Y., Tokunaga, M., Moriyama, M., Kinoshita, H., Nakamura, Y. Beneficial effects of troglitazone on neutrophil dysfunction in multiple low-dose streptozotocin-induced diabetic mice. *Clin. Exp. Immun*. 2004;137:263–71.

[110] Howarth, C. F., Qureshi, A., Shahin, A., Lukic, M. L. Effects of single high-dose and multiple low-dose streptozotocin on contraction and intracellular Ca2+ in ventricular myocytes from diabetes resistant and susceptible rats. *Mol. Cel. Biochem*. 2005;269: 103–8.

[111] Gao, Z., Leng, S., Lu, F., Xie, M., Xu, L., Wang, K. Effect of berberine on expression of hepatocyte nuclear factor-4α in rats with fructose-induced insulin resistance. *J. Huazhong Univ. Sci. Techn*. 2008;28:261–5.

[112] Hennig, B., Dupont, J. Lipoprotein lipid and protein responses to dietary fat and diabetes in rats. *J. Nutr*. 1983;113:1984-94.

[113] Tepper, B. J., Friedman, M. I. Diabetes and a high-fat/low-carbohydrate diet enhance the acceptability of oil emulsions to rats. *Physiol. Behav*. 1989;45:717-21.

[114] Moore, M. C., Cherrington, A. D., Mann, S. L., Davis, S. N. Acute fructose administration decreases the glycemic response to an oral glucose tolerance test in normal adults. *J. Clin. Endocrin. Metab*., 2000;85:4515–9.

[115] Masiello, P., Broca, C., Gross, R., Roye, M., Manteghetti, M., Hillaire-Buys, D., Novelli, M., Ribes, G. Experimental NIDDM: development of a new model in adult rats administered streptozotocin and nicotinamide. *Diabetes*. 1998;47:224-9.

[116] De Rijk, E. P., van Esch, E., Flik, G. Pregnancy dating in the rat: placental morphology and maternal blood parameters. *Toxicol. Pathol*. 2002;30:271-82.

[117] Damasceno, D. C., Kiss, A. C., Sinzato, Y. K., de Campos, K. E., Rudge, M. V., Calderon, I. M., Volpato, G. T. Maternal-fetal outcome, lipid profile and oxidative stress of diabetic rats neonatally exposed to streptozotocin. *Exp. Clin. Endoc. Diab*. 2011; 119:408-13.

[118] Blondel, O., Bailbe, D., Portha, B. Relation of insulin deficiency to impaired insulin action in NIDDM adult rats given streptozocin as neonates. *Diabetes*. 1989;38:610–7.

[119] Blondel, O., Bailbe, D., Portha, B. Insulin resistance in rats with non-insulin-dependent diabetes induced by neonatal (5 days) streptozotocin: evidence for reversal following phlorizin treatment. *Metabolism*. 1990;39:787–93.

[120] Eriksson, U., Dahlstrom, E., Larsson, K. S., Hellerstrom, C. Increased incidence of congenital malformations in the offspring of diabetic rats and their prevention by maternal insulin therapy. *Diabetes*. 1982;31:1–6.

[121] Caluwaerts, S., Holemans, K., van Bree, R., Verhaeghe, J., Van Assche, F. A. Is low-dose streptozotocin in rats an adequate model for gestational diabetes mellitus? *J. Soc. Gynecol. Investig*. 2003;10:216-21.

[122] Heinze, E., Vetter, U. Skeletal growth of fetuses from streptozotocin diabetic rat mothers: in vivo and in vitro studies. *Diabetologia*. 1987; 30:100-3.

[123] Lima, P. H., Sinzato, Y. K., Gelaleti, R. B., Calderon, I. M., Rudge, M. V., Damasceno, D. C. Genotoxicity evaluation in severe or mild diabetic pregnancy in laboratory animals. *Exp. Clin. End. Diab*. 2012;120:303-7.

[124] López-Soldado, I., Herrera, E. Different diabetogenic response to moderate doses of streptozotocin in pregnant rats, and its long-term consequences in the offspring. *Exp. Diabesity Res*. 2003;4:107-18.

[125] Gelardi, N. L., Cha, C. J., Oh, W. Glucose metabolism in adipocytes of obese offspring of mild hyperglycemic rats. *Pediatr. Res*. 1990;28:641-5.

In: Streptozotocin: Uses, Mechanism of Action and Side Effects ISBN: 978-1-63117-255-7
Editor: Elizabeth L. Gauthier 

*Chapter 5*

# MATRIX METALLOPROTEASES IN STREPTOZOTOCIN MODEL OF DIABETES MELLITUS

***Giovani B. Peres*[1], *Miriam G. Jasiulionis*[2] *and Yara M. Michelacci*[1]***

[1]Departamento de Bioquímica, and [2]Departamento de Farmacologia, Escola Paulista de Medicina, UNIFESP, São Paulo, SP, Brazil

## ABSTRACT

*M*atrix *m*etallo*p*roteases (MMPs) are a family of metal ion-dependent extracellular matrix (ECM) degrading enzymes that play crucial roles in tissue remodeling and repair, and may be involved in the development and progression of diabetic complications.

The most frequent complications in diabetes mellitus are consequences of macro- and microangiopathies, which affect many organs and tissues. Diabetic macroangiopathy manifests as an atherosclerosis-like condition, characterized by formation of plaques that follows an accelerated course, and diabetic microangiopathy is characterized by progressive arteriolosclerosis and interstitial fibrosis, with ECM accumulation and changes in its quality, as well as basement membrane thickening. These are structural hallmarks in all organs affected by diabetic complications, and may occur in response to insults such as hyperglycemia and hypertension.

A few examples illustrate the relevance of MMPs in diabetic complications: regarding cardiovascular system, it was shown that inhibition of MMP-2 and MMP-9 ameliorates cardiovascular dysfunction, becoming a possible therapeutic target; in diabetic brain, increased MMP activities (especially MMP-9) were reported, possibly contributing to blood-brain barrier degradation and cognitive impairment; increased MMP-9 occurs in diabetic skin, especially around wounds, and its expression was inhibited by siRNA, maybe providing a new therapeutic approach for diabetic skin wounds; MMP-2 and MMP-9 activities were shown to be increased in sera and placentas of diabetic rats, and both decreased when the animals were treated with dietary olive and safflower oils; in diabetic nephropathy, the accumulation of ECM leads to

* Corresponding author: Yara M. Michelacci, PhD; Disciplina de Biologia Molecular – Departamento de Bioquímica; Escola Paulista de Medicina – UNIFESP; Rua Três de Maio, 100; 04044-020 – São Paulo –SP– Brazil; E-mail: yara.bioq@epm.br; Telephone: 55-11-5576-4438, ext. 1187; FAX: 55-11-5573-6407.

glomerulosclerosis, interstitial fibrosis, tubular atrophy, and finally renal failure, and MMPs may be involved; recent evidences suggest that diabetes is a risk factor for the development of progressive liver disease, including non-alcoholic steatohepatitis, cirrhosis, and primary liver cancer. *In vitro* studies have shown that high glucose concentration can alter the expression of some MMPs (and also their endogenous inhibitors, TIMPs), and this effect might be mediated by connective tissue growth factor.

Hence, the aim of the present paper is to set the stage for a better understanding of the role of MMPs in streptozotocin-induced diabetes mellitus, focusing the main targets of diabetic complications: heart, brain, skin, uterus, kidney, and liver. In addition to discussing the literature, unpublished results on kidney and liver are also given.

## INTRODUCTION

Proteases are ancient and efficient enzymes that catalyze a common chemical reaction: the hydrolysis of peptide bonds. These enzymes not only demolish unwanted proteins, but also accomplish very specific proteolytic processing, leading to the formation of new peptides and proteins, with different biological activities. Thus, proteases influence multiple biological activities, such as DNA replication and transcription, cell proliferation and differentiation, wound healing, hemostasis, blood coagulation, inflammation, immunology, autophagy, and apoptosis. Based on the mechanisms of catalysis, proteases are classified into six distinct groups: aspartic, cysteine, glutamic, serine, threonine, and metalloproteases (López-Otín & Bond, 2008).

Among metalloproteases, some are matrix metalloproteases (MMPs), a family of extracellular endopeptidases that depend on calcium and zinc for their catalytic activities. They are active at neutral pH, and act primarily on extracellular matrix (ECM) components, regulating developmental and physiological events. MMPs are synthesized as pro-enzymes, and processed to the active form by the removal of an amino-terminal pro-peptide. Their main endogenous inhibitors are the *t*issue *i*nhibitors of *m*etallo*p*roteases, TIMPs.

The first MMP was discovered back in 1962, by Jerome Gross and Charles M. Lapiere (Gross & Lapiere, 1962), as a collagenolytic activity present during tadpole tail digestion. Nowadays, almost 30 MMPs have been described in humans, assigned to eight distinct classes, according to their structures: five classes are secreted, and three are membrane-bound (Egeblad & Werb, 2002).

All human MMPs share common structural domains (Figure 1), which include: (a) the signal peptide or pre-domain, consisting of 17-20 amino acid residues, rich in hydrophobic amino acids, that directs them for endoplasmic reticulum; (b) the pro-peptide domain, about 80 amino acids long, with a zinc-interacting thiol group (SH) that maintains MMPs as zymogens; (c) the catalytic domain of about 160-170 amino acids, with a zinc-binding motif containing three histidine residues; (d) the C-terminal hemopexin-like domain, consisting of about 210 amino acids, with a disulphite bond that orient the domain towards the formation of a four-bladed propeller structure. Additionally, the catalytic domain of MMPs-2 and 9 contain three fibronectin-type II motifs that interact with collagens and gelatins, while other domains may also be present: a furin-cleavage site insert in pro-peptide domain, a hinge region that links the catalytic domain to the hemopexin-like domain, and transmembrane insertion extensions (in membrane type MMPs, named MT-MMPs). Table 1 summarizes human MMPs arranged by structural classes and subgroups.

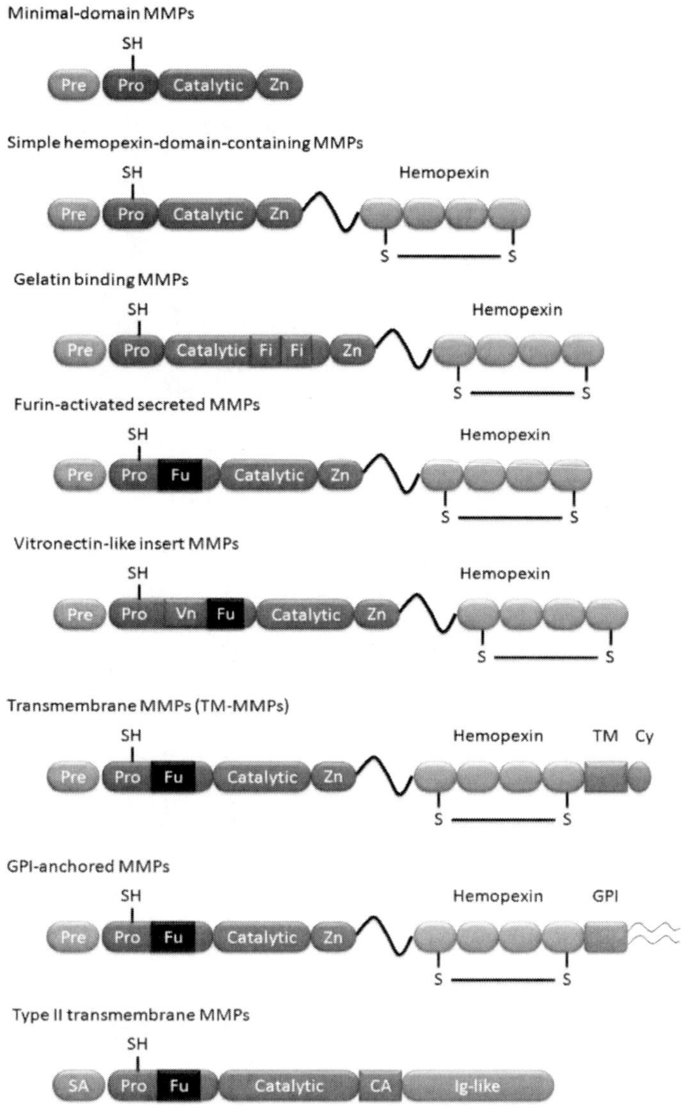


Figure 1. Structural domains of matrix metalloproteases (MMPs). MMPs are assigned to eight classes on the basis of their structural characteristics, five of which are secreted and three are membrane-type MMPs (MT-MMPs). From the N-terminus, MMPs contain the *Pre*, pre-peptide; *Pro*, pro-domain containing a highly conserved sequence with a cysteine thiol group (*SH*) that interacts with zinc, and maintains the enzyme as inactive zymogen; *Catalytic* domain with a zinc (*Zn*) binding site; Hemopexin-like domain (*Hemopexin*) linked to the catalytic domain by a *Hinge* (~), which mediates interactions with tissue inhibitors of metalloproteases, cell surface molecules and substrates. The first and the last hemopexin-like repeats are linked by a disulphite bond (*S-S*). A recognition motif for intracellular furin-like serine proteases (*Fu*) may be present between the pro-peptide and the catalytic domain, and the gelatin-binding MMPs contain inserts that resemble collating-binding repeats of fibronectina (*Fi*). Other inserts are present in MT-MMPs: a single-span transmembrane domain (*TM*), a very short cytoplasmic domain (*Cy*), and the glycosylphosphatidylinositol anchor (*GPI*). In Type II MT-MMPs, an N-terminal signal anchor (*SA*), an unique cysteine array (*CA*) and an immunoglobulin-like (*Ig-like*) domain are also present. Adapted from Egeblad & Werb (2002).

The main function of MMPs is presumed to be ECM remodeling, but today it is clear that MMPs also influence cellular function in several ways: (1) allowing cell migration through ECM digestion; (2) affecting cell behavior through changes in the extracellular micro-environment; (3) modulating the activity of biological molecules by direct cleavage, release from stores, or control of the activity of inhibitors (Vu & Werb, 2000).

In diabetes mellitus, fibrosis may occur in many tissues as a response to insults such as hyperglycemia and hypertension, and MMPs may be involved in the development and progression of diabetic complications. Fibrosis is characterized by ECM accumulation and changes in its quality, as well as basement membrane thickening, which are structural hallmarks in all target organs of diabetic complications (Ban and Twigg, 2008). It is widely accepted that the onset and progression of diabetic complications is a consequence of macro- or microangiopathy (Schalkwijk & Stehouwer, 2005), which are strongly linked to the sustained hyperglycemia (The Diabetes Control and Complications Trial Research Group, 1993; UK Prospective Diabetes Study - UKPDS Group, 1998; Torffvit, 2003; Yan et al., 2003), maybe mediated by *a*dvanced *g*lycation *e*ndproduts (AGEs) (Goh & Cooper, 2008), formed by non-enzymatic glycation of proteins, lipids, and nucleic acids.

High glucose concentration and AGEs can alter the expression of some MMPs and TIMPs (McLennan et al., 1998; DeGroot et al., 2001; Zhang et al., 2011), and this could be one of the mechanisms leading to the complications in diabetes mellitus.

The present paper discusses the relevance of MMPs for diabetic complications affecting different organs and systems in the streptozotocin-induced type 1 diabetes mellitus.

## CARDIOVASCULAR SYSTEM

Diabetic cardiomyopathy is one common complication in people with diabetes, leading to heart failure (Avogaro et al., 2004), with ventricular dilation, myocyte hypertrophy, interstitial fibrosis and presence of a diastolic dysfunction (Severson, 2004). Microangiopathy, characterized by subendothelial and endothelial fibrosis in coronary microvasculature of the heart, is one of the causes of diabetic heart failure. Hyperglycemia is considered one of the factors that lead to endothelial impairment.

One of the consequences of high glucose concentration is the formation of AGEs. Structural components of the extracellular matrix are highly susceptible to glycation because of their low turnover rates (Vlassara et al., 1992), causing aberrant cross links and its complications. Extracellular matrix AGEs also interfere with cell-matrix interactions, modifying cell adhesion and signaling (Haitoglou et al., 1992). Binding of AGEs to cell surface receptors, such as RAGE (Yan et al., 2010) and AGE-R1 (Lu et al., 2004), activate cell signaling pathways that modulate gene expression, lead to generation of free radicals (Schmidt et al., 1999), and activate inflammatory pathways, both in tissue cells and in macrophages. RAGE deficiency attenuates the development of atherosclerosis in diabetes, indicating that RAGE plays a central role in this process (Soro-Paavonen et al., 2008). Furthermore, the binding of AGEs to extracellular proteins promotes fibrosis (Charonis et al., 1990). In fact, a major source of increased myocardial stiffness is cross linking between AGEs and collagen.

**Table 1. Human matrix metalloproteases (MMPs)[1]**

| MMP designation | Structural class | Common name | Substrates |
|---|---|---|---|
| **Collagenases** | | | |
| MMP-1 | Simple hemopexin domain | Collagenase-1 | Col I, II, III, VII, VIII, X, gelatin |
| MMP-8 | Simple hemopexin domain | Collagenase-2 | Col I, II, III, VII, VIII, X, gelatin, aggrecan |
| MMP-13 | Simple hemopexin domain | Collagenase-3 | Col I, II, III, VII, VIII, X, gelatin |
| **Gelatinases** | | | |
| MMP-2 | Gelatin binding | Gelatinase A | Col I, II, III, VII, VIII, X, gelatin |
| MMP-9 | Gelatin binding | Gelatinase B | Col IV, V, gelatin |
| **Stromelysins** | | | |
| MMP-3 | Simple hemopexin domain | Stromelysin-1 | Col II, IV, IX, X, XI, gelatin |
| MMP-10 | Simple hemopexin domain | Stromelysin-2 | Col IV, elastin, fibronectin, laminin |
| MMP-11 | Furin-activated and secreted | Stromelysin-3 | Col IV, aggrecan, fibronectin, gelatin |
| **MMP designation** | **Structural class** | **Common name** | **Substrates** |
| **Matrilysins** | | | |
| MMP-7 | Minimal domain | Matrilysin | Col IV, fibronectin, gelatin, laminin, tenascin |
| MMP-26 | Minimal domain | Matrilysin-2 | Fibrinogen, fibronectin, gelatin |
| **MT-MMPs** | | | |
| MMP-14 | Transmembrane | MT1-MMP | Fibronectin, gelatin, laminin |
| MMP-15 | Transmembrane | MT2-MMP | Fibronectin, gelatin, laminin |
| MMP-16 | Transmembrane | MT3-MMP | Fibronectin, gelatin, laminin |
| MMP-17 | GPI-linked | MT4-MMP | Fibrin, fibrinogen |
| MMP-24 | Transmembrane | MT5-MMP | Fibronectin, gelatin, laminin |
| MMP-25 | GPI-linked | MT6-MMP | Gelatin |
| **Other** | | | |
| MMP-12 | Simple hemopexin domain | Metalloelastase | Col IV, elastin, fibronectin |
| MMP-19 | Simple hemopexin domain | RASI-1 | Aggrecan, Col IV, elastin, fibrillin, gelatin |
| MMP-20 | Simple hemopexin domain | Enamelysin | Aggrecan |
| MMP-21 | Vitronectin-like insert | XMMP | Aggrecan |
| MMP-23 | Type II transmembrane | Cys-array MMP | Casein, fibronectin, gelatin |
| MMP-27 | Simple hemopexin domain | CMMP | Collagen |
| MMP-28 | Furin-activated and secreted | Epilysin | E-cadherin (regulate epithelial–mesenchymal transition) |

[1] According to Keeling and Herrera (2008) and Spinale (2013).

Although many cells are able to regulate their transport of glucose, maintaining internal glucose concentrations constant even under hyperglycemia, some cells, such as endothelial and mesangial cells, cannot do this efficiently, and are susceptible to intracellular high glucose concentrations and AGE formation (Kaiser et al., 1993; Heilig et al., 1995). This is important because glucose-derived intermediates (such as glyceraldehyde-3-phosphate, dihydroxyacetonephosphate, glyoxal and methylglyoxal) and intracellular sugars (such as ribose) form glycated proteins faster than glucose itself (Thornalley, 2005). Intracellular AGEs are implicated in the activation of signaling pathways (Giardino et al., 1994), and in the cross linking of proteins that form intracellular aggregates, resistant to the action of proteases (Brownlee, 1995).

It was shown that streptozotocin is able to induce diabetic cardiomyopathy (Li et al., 2012), and treatment with either alpha-lipoic acid or aminoguanidine decreased collagen deposition and enhanced extracellular matrix degradation (Li et al., 2012; Vadla & Vellaichamy, 2012). Uemura et al., (2001) have shown increased expression and activity of MMP-9, but not MMP-2, in bovine aortic endothelial cells chronically exposed to high glucose. Similar results were obtained in *in vivo* experiments, with streptozotocin-diabetic rats: increased MMP-9 was observed in the left ventricle of hyperglycemic rats, but not in diabetic rats with good glycemic control (Sung et al., 2009). Moreover, it seems that oxidative stress plays an important role, since treatment with antioxidants significantly reduced the enhanced MMP-9. Treatment with minocycline, a second generation tetracycline able to suppress oxidative stress (Sinha-Hikim et al., 2011), decreased collagen, MMP-2 and MMP-9 in aorta of streptozotocin-diabetic rats (Bhatt & Veeranjaneyulu, 2012).

On the other hand, decreased activity of MMP-2, and increased expression of TIMP-2 (10-fold) were observed in streptozotocin-induced cardiac fibrosis in rats (Van Linthoud et al., 2008). Also in minipigs, streptozotocin-induced diabetes led to increased TIMP-1 and decreased MMP-2 and MMP-9 activities in aorta and myocardium, indicating that MMP-TIMP dysregulation is associated with cardiac dysfunction and cardiovascular fibrosis in diabetes (Lu et al., 2008).

## Brain

Diabetes mellitus is associated with peripheral microvascular complications and increased risk of neurological events. Among the manifestations of brain damage caused by diabetes are blood-brain barrier disruption and edema. MMP activity is increased in the plasma of diabetic patients, and it is a known mediator of blood-brain barrier degradation. Hawkins et al., (2007) have shown that diabetes increases the blood-brain barrier permeability via loss of tight junction proteins. This is possibly due to increased plasma MMP activities, which are implicated in the degradation of tight junction proteins, leading to increased blood-brain barrier permeability. It was also shown that hyperglycemia increases both oxidative stress and MMP-9 activity, exacerbating blood-brain barrier dysfunction after ischemia/reperfusion injury (Kamada et al., 2007).

Furthermore, diabetes may induce cognitive decline. It was recently shown that rats that developed cognitive deficit presented increased expression of MMP-9 and NF-κB in hippocampus. Inhibition of NF-κB by pyrrolidine dithiocarbamate returned NF-κB to basal levels and improved the diabetic-associated behavioral deficit, but did not normalize the MMP-9 expression (Zhao et al., 2013), which remained high. High MMP-9 may contribute to the blood-brain barrier degradation, and cognitive impairment. In fact, Oltman et al., (2011) have shown that treatment of streptozotocin-diabetic rats with inhibitors of neutral endopeptidases and angiotensin converting enzyme improved both neural and vascular functions.

## Skin and Wound Healing

Diabetes mellitus frequently leads to delayed wound healing. Rats with type I streptozotocin-induced diabetes mellitus also exhibited slower wound healing, and higher dermal collagenase activity (Mohanam & Bose, 1983). This is probably due to increased expression (both mRNA and protein) of MMP-9, with decreased expression of TIMP-1 (Yang et al., 2009).

Also *in vitro*, skin explants from streptozotocin-diabetic rats have shown increased levels of MMP-9 and MMP-13 (4- and 10-fold, respectively), in comparison to controls. Treatment with retinoic acid, the active form of vitamin A, reduced MMPs by 50-75%, and increased collagen synthesis (Varani et al., 2002). Furthermore, wrinkles were observed in the skin of streptozotocin-induced diabetic rats, similar to those observed in vitamin A-deficient rats. The activities of MMP-2 and hyaluronidase (Hyase) were found to be increased in the skin of these animals, but decreased upon treatment with retinoic acid. Blood retinol levels were lower than normal in diabetic rats. These results indicate a possible relationship between streptozotocin-induced diabetes and vitamin A-deficiency on MMP and Hyase in skin, and that vitamin A might be a regulator of ECM-degrading enzymes (Takahashi & Takasu, 2011). The expression of MMP-9 was inhibited by small interfering RNA (siRNA), maybe providing a new therapeutic approach for diabetic skin wound (Xie et al., 2012).

Concerning the relationship between AGEs and matrix degradation by MMPs, a strong correlation was observed between collagen glycation and collagenase activity (Hennessey et al., 1990): the higher blood glucose, the higher collagenase activity, and consequently the lower wound collagen content. It was also shown that the activity of MMP-2, as well as the protein levels of MMP-3 and MMP-13, was increased in diabetic mice, treated or not with aminoguanidine, an AGE-formation blocker. Nevertheless, collagenolysis was decreased in untreated diabetic mice, and treatment of diabetic mice with aminoguanidine restored collagenolysis to normal levels, indicating that AGEs impair extracellular matrix degradation (Tamarat et al., 2003).

## PLACENTA

MMPs are responsible for the remodeling of the uterine extracellular matrix during embryo implantation. Increased levels and activity of MMP-2 were detected in streptozotocin-induced diabetic rats, in comparison to controls. The uterine enzymatic activity in diabetic animals decreased in the presence of NOS inhibitor, and was enhanced in presence of a generating ROS system (Pustovrh et al., 2002). Also, MMPs are involved in placental remodeling throughout pregnancy. MMP-2 and MMP-9 were found to be increased in diabetic placenta, in both maternal and fetal sides. Moreover, in both sides of the diabetic placenta, nitrate/nitrite concentrations (which indicate NO production) were also increased (Pustovrh et al., 2005). The same authors have also shown that addition of 15deoxy Delta (12,14) prostaglandin J-2 (15dPGJ(2)), a natural ligand of the peroxisome proliferator activated receptor (PPAR) gamma, reduced the increased activities of MMP-2 and MMP-9 in diabetic placenta. On the contrary, TIMP-3 levels, which were decreased in diabetic placentas, were increased by 15dPGJ(2) (Pustovrh et al., 2009). Also, diet supplements with olive and safflower oil, which are enriched in natural PPAR ligands (Martinez et al., 2012), and with folic acid (Higa et al., 2012) are able to prevent MMP-2 and MMP-9 overactivities in the placenta of diabetic rats, protecting the embryo from diabetic-induced damage.

## KIDNEY AND LIVER

In diabetic nephropathy, renal hypertrophy and accumulation of ECM proteins are well recognized features. Regardless of the factors that initiate the renal injury, the progression of renal disease ultimately results in the accumulation of ECM, leading to glomerulosclerosis, interstitial fibrosis, tubular atrophy, and finally renal failure (Williams et al., 2011). This might result of increased protein synthesis (Barac-Nieto et al., 1991), or decreased degradation (Shechter et al., 1994), or both. MMPs may be involved.

In 2005, it was shown that dextran sulfate administered to diabetic rats accumulated in liver and kidney (de Lima et al., 2005), and this could be due to malfunction of the lysosomal pathway for digestion of macromolecule. Recently, decreased activities of lysosomal cathepsins (especially cathepsin B) and glycosidases (especially β-glucuronidase) were reported in the kidney of diabetic rats (type 1) during the early stages of the disease (10 and 30 days) (Peres et al., 2013a). This is in agreement with results obtained by others (Mohanam & Bose, 1983), and could be one of the mechanisms leading to ECM accumulation in diabetic nephropathy.

MMPs are also possible candidates for matrix remodeling in diabetic nephropathy and liver disease. Decreased collagenase activity in kidney of streptozotocin-diabetic rats in comparison to controls has been previously reported (Lubec et al., 1982; Mohanam & Bose, 1983), while similar activities were observed in liver. In contrast, skin and serum collagenase activities were increased (Mohanam & Bose, 1983).

*In vitro* studies have shown that MMP-2 activity was decreased in rat mesangial cells cultured in presence of high glucose concentrations (Kitamura et al., 1992; Leehey et al., 1995), while TIMP was increased (Kitamura et al., 1992; Singh et al., 2001). This effect seems to be mediated by transforming growth factor β1 (TGF-β1), which was increased in presence of high glucose (Singh et al., 2001).

Decreased MMP activities were also observed in isolated glomerulus from streptozotocin-diabetic rats, and this could contribute to mesangial expansion and glomerular basement membrane thickening. A marked decrease was observed for MMPs on the 4th day of diabetes, and MMP levels remained low for five weeks, irrespective of insulin-treatment (Reckelhoff et al., 1993; Schaefer et al., 1994; Song et al., 1999). Nakamura et al (1994) have shown that the expression (mRNA) of MMP-1 and -3 was decreased in the glomeruli of diabetic rats, but the expression of MMP-2 did not vary, and MMP-9 was not detected. In contrast, other authors reported decreased expression of MMP-2 in diabetic rat kidney (Wu et al., 1997), and in long term diabetes (six months), decreased mRNA and activity of MMP-9 were reported, while MMP-2 mRNA was increased and its activity was decreased (McLennan et al., 2002). Two to eight weeks after streptozotocin administration, decreased expression of MMP-2 in the glomeruli and increased expression in the interstitium were reported, while the expression of MMP-9 did not vary in diabetic kidney. Increased expression of collagen type-IV occurred both in the glomeruli and the interstitium (Dong et al., 2004). In contrast, the expression of TIMP-1 mRNA was found to be increased in diabetic kidney (Nakamura et al., 1994; Wu et al., 1997; McLennan et al., 2002), and it seems that the imbalance between MMPs and TIMPs may contribute to the diabetic nephropathy (Han et al., 2006; Sun et al., 2006).

Concerning the liver, recent evidences suggest that diabetes is a risk factor for the development of progressive liver disease, including non-alcoholic steatohepatitis, cirrhosis, and primary liver cancer (Loria et al., 2013). It was shown that, also in liver, the activities of lysosomal cathepsins were decreased in diabetes, although the expression and activities of glycosidases did not vary, suggesting modulation of gene expressions and changes in enzyme activities, but not general lysosomal failure (Peres et al., 2013b).

Since different results were reported by different authors, depending on the experimental design, period of diabetes, streptozotocin dose, and glucose levels, we decided to investigate the expression of MMPs in kidney and liver of diabetic rats, under the same conditions used to measure lysosomal enzymes (10 and 30 days after streptozotocin administration).

The gelatinolytic activities of liver and kidney from normal (NL) and diabetic (DM) rats, both on the 10th and 30th days after diabetes induction, are shown in Figure 2. It is evident that the gelatinolytic activities were much higher in kidney than in liver, and the most visible bands were of high molecular weight (>100 kDa). Better resolution was obtained with lower amounts of kidney extracts (10 μg of protein) and gradient polyacrylamide gel (6-20%), but again the main bands were of high molecular weight. The bands corresponding to MMP-2 (67-72 kDa) and MMP-9 (89-92 kDa) did not appear. It is possible that the high molecular weight gelatinolytic activities are macromolecular, heteropolymeric complexes of MMP-2 and MMP-9 (Hussain et al., 2010).

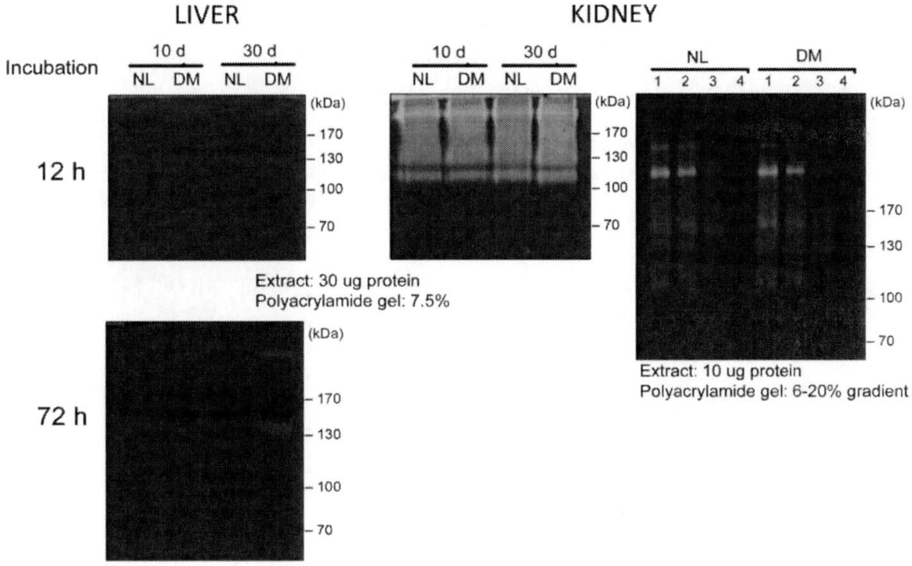


Figure 2. Gelatinolytic activities in liver and kidney of diabetic (DM) and normal (NL) rats. Liver and kidney extracts (either 30 μg or 10 μg of protein, as indicated) from four animals of each group were pooled, and aliquots were submitted to SDS-PAGE in either 7.5% or 4-20% gradient gels, copolymerized with 1 mg/ml gelatin, as previously described (Shapiro et al., 2001). After the run, SDS was removed by washing the polyacrylamide gel with 2% Triton X-100, and then the gels were transferred to 50 mM Tris-HCl buffer, pH 8.2, containing 5 mM $CaCl_2$ and 0.5 μM $ZnCl_2$. After 12 h (kidney and liver) or 72 h (liver) incubations, the gels were stained by Coomasie Blue. After destaining, gelatinolytic activities appeared as clear halos. To test for the presence of other proteases, before the electrophoresis, aliquots of the pooled kidney extracts were incubated with the following inhibitors (15 min in ice bath): (1) no inhibitor; (2) 5 μM E64 (irreversible inhibitor of cysteine-proteases); (3) 2 mM ortho-phenanthroline (zinc chelator); (4) 10 mM ethylenediaminetetraacetic acid, EDTA (metal chelator, including calcium and zinc).

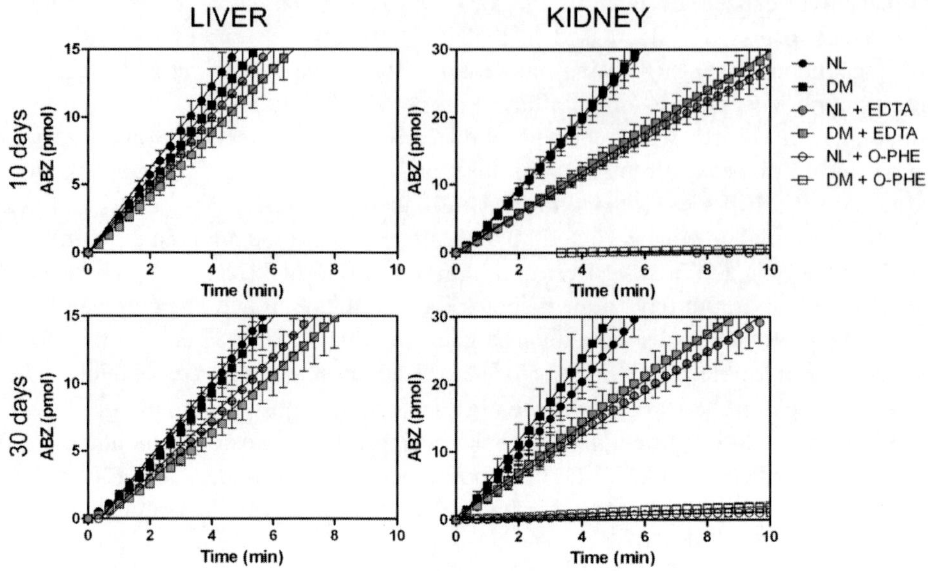


Figure 3. Kinetics of metalloprotease in liver and kidney extracts of normal (NL) and streptozotocin-diabetic (DM) rats. Tissue extracts (30 μg of protein from kidney, and 60 μg of protein from liver, n=30) were pre-incubated at 37°C for 30 seconds in Tris-HCl buffer, pH 8.2, containing 5 μM E64 and 1 mM PMSF, and then the substrate Abz-KLFSSKQ-EDDnp was added (10 μM, final concentration). Incubation mixtures (1 ml, final volume) were maintained at 37°C. The spectrofluorometer was adjusted to $\lambda_{ex}$ = 320 nm e $\lambda_{em}$ = 420 nm, and the fluorescence was measured every second. Incubations were also performed in presence of metalloprotease inhibitors: 10 mM EDTA and 2 mM orto-phenanthroline.

E64, which is a cysteine-protease inhibitor, had no effect upon kidney gelatinolytic activities, while in presence of either ortho-phenanthroline or EDTA (metal chelators) all gelatinolytic activities were inhibited, indicating that they are metalloproteases. In liver, gelatinolytic activities were much lower, and only a ~140 kDa band was observed after 72 h incubations (Figure 2). MMP activities measured by fluorometric assays[1] were also unaltered in diabetes (Figure 3 and Figure 4).

The expression of MMP-2 and MMP-9 (mRNA, measured by qPCR)[2] was decreased in diabetic liver and kidney (Figure 5), both 10 and 30 days after streptozotocin administration. Nevertheless, the amounts of MMP-2 and MMP-9 proteins (Western blotting, MW 72 kDa

[1] Fluorometric assays were performed by *f*luorescence *r*esonance *e*nergy *t*ransfer – FRET – based on the family of synthetic peptides Abz-KLXSSKQ-EDDnp (X = D, R, Y ou F) as substrates. Incubations were performed at 37°C in quartz cuvetes containing 50 mM Tris-HCl buffer, pH 8.2, protease inhibitors 5 μM E64 (irreversible inhibitor of cysteine-proteases), and 1 mM phenylmethylsulfonyl fluoride (PMSF, inhibitor of serine-proteases), tissue extracts (30 μg of protein for kidney and 60 μg of protein for liver), and then the substrate was added (10 μM, 1 ml final volume). The assays were also performed in presence of MMP inhibitors: 10 mM ethylenediamine tetraacetic acid (EDTA, calcium chelator) or 2 mM ortho-phenanthroline (zinc chelator). The peptides formed upon substrate digestion were identified by HPLC.

[2] The primers used for real time qPCR were: MMP-2, forward 5' GGCACCACCGAGGATTATGACC 3', and reverse, 5' GTGAAGGGGAAGACACATGGGG 3'; MMP-9, forward 5' CACCACTAAAGGTCGCT CGGATG 3', and reverse, 5' GGAAGACGCACATCTCTCCTGC 3'. Housekeeping genes: β-actin, forward 5' GGATGACGATATCGCTGCGCT 3', and reverse 5' CTGACCCATACCCACCATCACAC 3', and ribosomal protein 29S, forward 5' GTCAGTACGCGAAGGACATAGGC 3', and reverse 5' CAGGGTAGACAGTTGGTTTCATTGGG 3'. Relative gene expression was calculated by the $2^{-\Delta\Delta C_T}$ method developed by Livak & Schmittgen (2001).

and 92 kDa, respectively) did not significantly vary in diabetes (Figure 6). MMP-2 and MMP-9 concentrations were much lower in liver than in kidney, but no detectable changes in protein amounts were observed in diabetic tissues, in comparison to matched controls.

Concerning MMPs that act on extracellular matrix proteins other than collagen, it was shown that MMP-7, which may play a role in fibronectin accumulation, was reduced by exposure of mesangial cells to AGEs. Both the MMP-7 increase and the fibronectin accumulation were attenuated by aminoguanidine, an inhibitor of glycation product formation (McLennan et al., 2007).

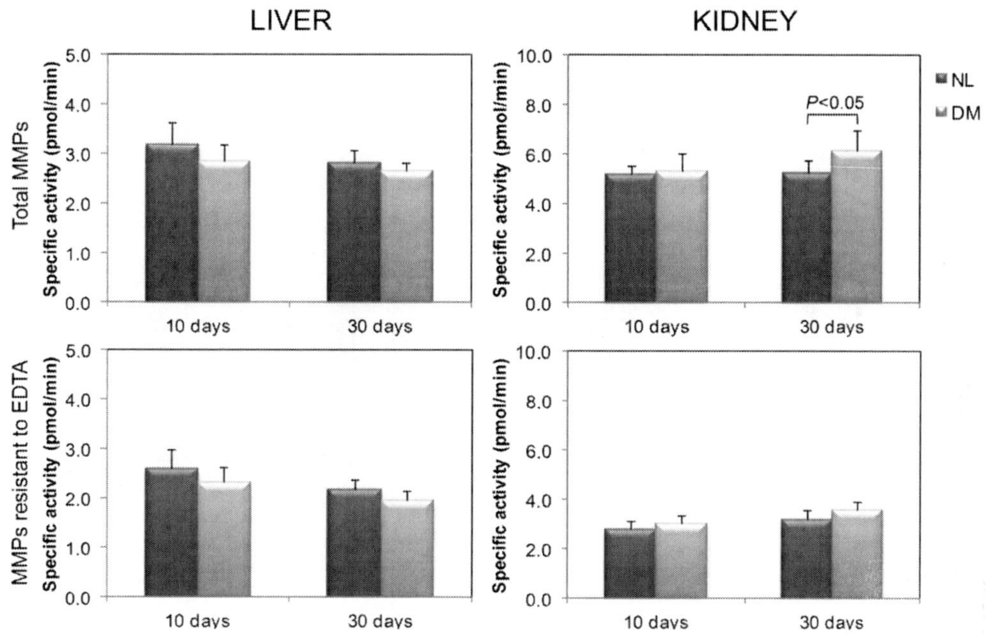


Figure 4. Specific activities of metalloproteases in diabetic (DM) and normal (NL) rat kidney and liver. The assays were performed as described in Figure 3, except that specific activities are shown (pmol/min/μg of protein). Data represents mean±standard deviation. Statistically significant differences between NL and DM are shown as p<0.05.

## CONCLUSION

Many of the complications that occur in human diabetes mellitus also occur in the streptozotocin-induced disease, indicating that this is a good model to investigate the macromolecules and enzymes involved in the onset and progression of these complications. The present paper focused on the expression and activities of matrix metalloproteases in streptozotocin-diabetes mellitus, in different organs and tissues, and it is clear that MMPs may be involved in diabetic complications. Changes in both the expression and the activities of these enzymes may be affected by high glucose and/or AGEs. So, MMPs and their endogenous inhibitors – TIMPs – may be important targets to control the onset and progression of diabetes mellitus complications.

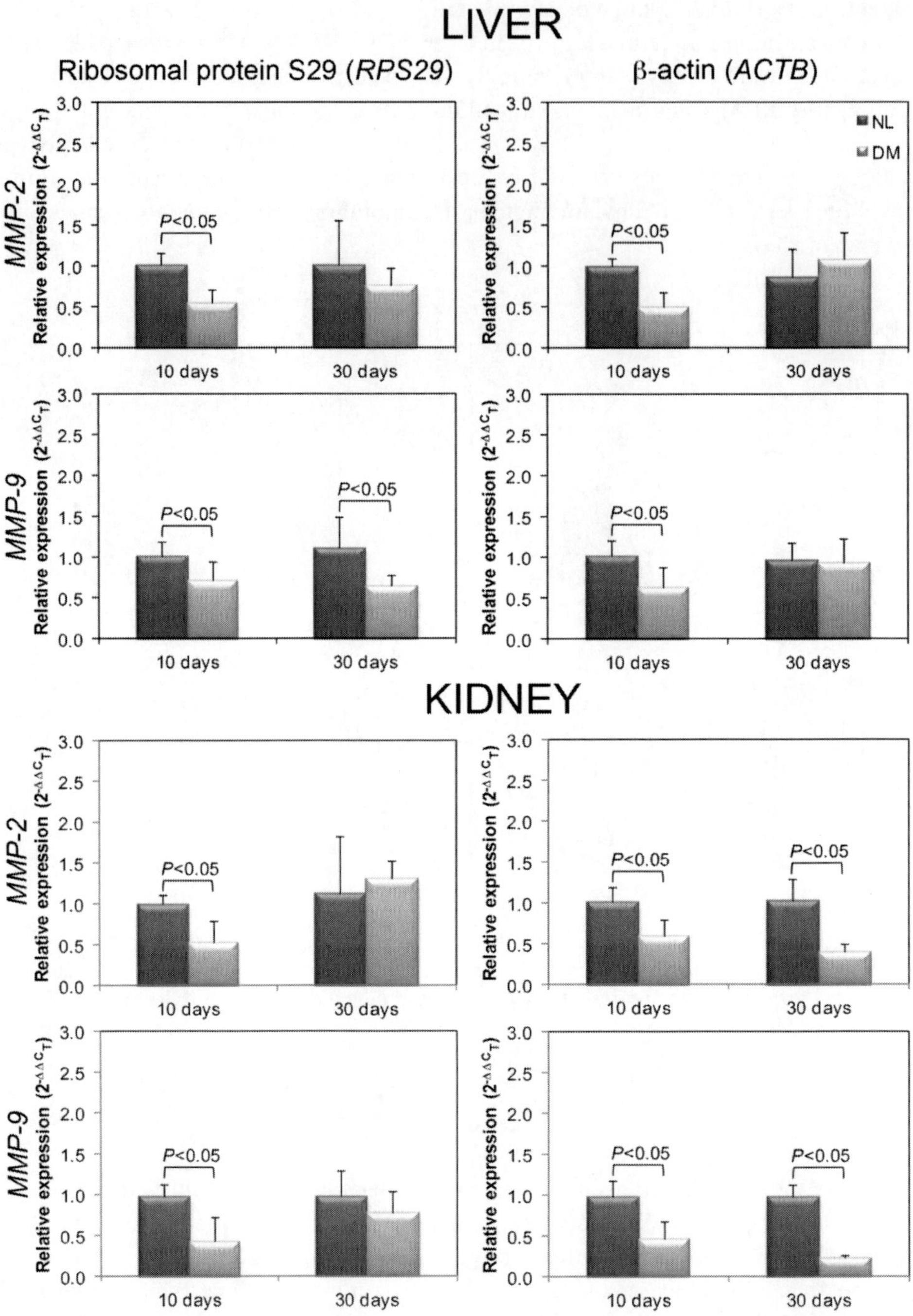


Figure 5. Expression (mRNA) of MMP-2 and MMP-9 in diabetic (DM) and normal (NL) rat liver and kidney. The expression of mRNA was normalized either by ribosomal protein S29 (*RPS29*) or β-actin (*ACTB*). Data represent mean±standard deviation (n=60). Statistically significant differences between NL and DM are shown as $p<0.05$.

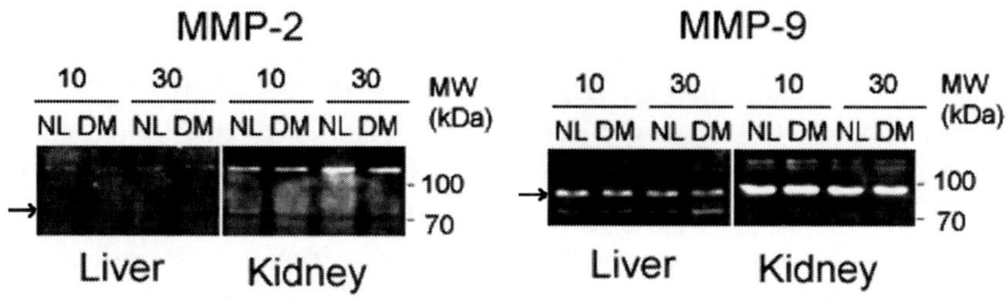


Figure 6. Representative Western blottings of MMP-2 and MMP-9 extracted from diabetic (DM) and normal (NL) rat liver and kidney. Tissue extracts (3-5 μl containing 30 μg of protein) were submitted to SDS-PAGE (7.5% acrylamide with 0.2% bisacrylamide). Proteins were transferred to nitrocellulose membranes, probed with either rabbit polyclonal anti-MMP-2 (Millipore AB19167, 1:500) or anti-MMP-9 (Millipore AB6001, 1:2000) antibodies. Specific bands were detected by secondary antibody (anti-rabbit IgG) conjugated with horseradish peroxidase (HRP) and ECL-chemiluminescent substrate. Images were obtained with MF-ChemiBIS gel documentation system. Each lane represents a pool of four animals of each group.

## ACKNOWLEDGEMENTS

The authors want to express their gratitude to Prof. Dr. Maria A. Juliano, who synthesized the substrates for MMPs, and permitted the use of her laboratory for the studies on enzyme kinetics. The authors also acknowledge the financial support of Fundação de Amparo à Pesquisa do Estado de São Paulo (FAPESP, grants #2013/07109-8, #2010/16022-5, and #2009/11817-2), São Paulo, SP, Brazil; Conselho Nacional de Desenvolvimento Científico e Tecnológico (CNPq, grant #308642/2010-4), Brasília, DF, Brazil; and Fundação Coordenação de Aperfeiçoamento de Pessoal de Nível Superior (CAPES), Brasília, SP, Brazil.

## REFERENCES

Avogaro, A., Vigili de Kreutzenberg, S., Negut, C., Tiengo, A. & Scognamiglio, R. (2004). Diabetic cardiomyopathy: a metabolic perspective. *Am. J. Cardiol.* 93, 13A–16A.

Ban, C. R. & Twigg, S. M. (2008). Fibrosis in diabetes complications: Pathogenic mechanisms and circulating and urinary markers. *Vasc. Health Risk Manag.* 4, 575-596.

Barac-Nieto, M., Liu, S. M. & Spitzer, A. (1991). Renal protein synthesis in diabetes mellitus: effects of insulin and insulin-like growth factor I. *Am. J. Kidney Dis.* 17, 658-660.

Bhatt, L. K. & Veeranjaneyulu, A. (2012). A therapeutic approach to treat cardiovascular dysfunction of diabetes. Exp. Toxicol. Pathol. 64, 847-853.

Brownlee, M. (1995). Advanced protein glycosylation in diabetes and aging. *Annu. Rev. Med.* 46, 223–234.

Charonis, A. S., Reger, L. A., Dege, J. E., Kouzi-Koliakos, K., Furcht, L. T., Wohlhueter, R. M. & Tsilibary, E. C. (1990). Laminin alterations after in vitro nonenzymatic glycosylation. *Diabetes* 39, 807–814.

de Lima, C. R., Aguiar, J. A. & Michelacci, Y. M. (2005). Reduced urinary excretion of sulfated polysaccharides in diabetic rats. *Biochim. Biophys. Acta* 1741, 30-41.

DeGroot. J., Verzijl, N., Wenting-Van Wijk, M. J., Bank, R. A., Lafeber, F. P., Bijlsma, J. W. & TeKoppele, J. M. (2001). Age-related decrease in susceptibility of human articular cartilage to matrix metalloproteinase-mediated degradation: the role of advanced glycation end products. *Arthritis Rheum.* 44, 2562-2571.

Dong, F. Q., Li, H., Cai, W. M., Tao, J., Li, Q., Ruan, Y., Zheng, F. P. & Zhang, Z. (2004). Effects of pioglitazone on expressions of matrix metalloproteinases 2 and 9 in kidneys of diabetic rats. *Chin Med J* (Engl) 117, 1040-1044.

Egeblad, M. & Werb, Z. (2002). New functions for the matrix metalloproteinases in cancer progression. *Nature Reviews* 2, 161-174.

Giardino, I., Edelstein, D. & Brownlee, M. (1994). Nonenzymatic glycosylation in vitro and in bovine endothelial cells alters basic fibroblast growth factor activity. A model for intracellular glycosylation in diabetes. *J. Clin. Invest.* 94, 110–117.

Goh, S. Y. & Cooper, M. E. (2008). Clinical review: the role of advanced glycation end products in progression and complications of diabetes. *J. Clin. Endocrinol. Metab.* 93, 1143–1152.

Gross, J. & Lapiere, C. M. (1962). Collagenolytic activity in amphibian tissues: a tissue culture assay. *Proc. Natl. Acad. Sci.* USA 48, 1014–1022.

Haitoglou, C. S., Tsilibary, E. C., Brownlee, M. & Charonis, A. S. (1992). Altered cellular interactions between endothelial cells and nonenzymatically glucosylated laminin/type IV collagen. *J. Biol. Chem.* 267, 12404–12407.

Han, S. Y., Jee, Y. H., Han, K. H., Kang, Y. S., Kim, H. K., Han, J. Y., Kim, Y. S. & Cha, D. R. (2006). An imbalance between matrix metalloproteinase-2 and tissue inhibitor of matrix metalloproteinase-2 contributes to the development of early diabetic nephropathy. *Nephrol. Dial. Transplant.* 21, 2406-2416.

Hawkins, B. T., Lundeen, T. F., Norwood, K. M., Brooks, H. L. & Egleton, R. D. (2007). Increased blood-brain barrier permeability and altered tight junctions in experimental diabetes in the rat: contribution of hyperglycaemia and matrix metalloproteinases. *Diabetologia* 50, 202-211.

Heilig, C. W., Concepcion, L. A., Riser, B. L., Freytag, S. O., Zhu, M. & Cortes, P. (1995). Overexpression of glucose transporters in rat mesangial cells cultured in a normal glucose milieu mimics the diabetic phenotype. *J. Clin. Invest.* 96, 1802–1814.

Hennessey, P. J., Ford, E. G., Black, C. T. & Andrassy, R. J. (1990). Wound collagenase activity correlates directly with collagen glycosylation in diabetic rats. *J. Pediatr. Surg.* 25, 75-78.

Higa, R., Kurtz, M., Mazzucco, M. B., Musikant, D., White, V. & Jawerbaum, A. (2012). Folic acid and safflower oil supplementation interacts and protects embryos from maternal diabetes-induced damage. *Mol. Hum. Reprod.* 18, 253-264.

Hussain, A. A., Lee, Y. & Marshall, J. (2010). High molecular weight gelatinase species of human Bruch's membrane: compositional analyses and age-related changes. *Invest. Ophth. Vis. Sci.* 51, 2363-2371.

Kaiser, N., Sasson, S., Feener, E. P., Boukobza-Vardi, N., Higashi, S., Moller, D. E., Davidheiser, S., Przybylski, R. J. & King, G. L. (1993). Differential regulation of glucose transport and transporters by glucose in vascular endothelial and smooth muscle cells. *Diabetes* 42, 80–89.

Kamada, H., Yu, F., Nito, C. & Chan, P. H. (2007). Influence of hyperglycemia on oxidative stress and matrix metalloproteinase-9 activation after focal cerebral ischemia/reperfusion in rats: relation to blood-brain barrier dysfunction. *Stroke* 38, 1044-1049.

Keeling, J. & Herrera, G. A. (2008) Human matrix metalloproteinases: characteristics and pathologic role in altering mesangial homeostasis Microsc. *Res. Tech.* 71, 371-379.

Kitamura, M., Kitamura, A., Mitarai, T., Maruyama, N., Nagasawa, R., Kawamura, T., Yoshida, H., Takahashi, T. & Sakai, O. (1992). Gene expression of metalloproteinase and its inhibitor in mesangial cells exposed to high glucose. *Biochem. Biophys. Res.* Commun. 185, 1048-1054.

Leehey, D. J., Song, R. H., Alavi, N. & Singh, A. K. (1995). Decreased degradative enzymes in mesangial cells cultured in high glucose media. *Diabetes* 44, 929-935.

Li, C. J., Lv, L., Li, H. & Yu, D. M. (2012). Cardiac fibrosis and dysfunction in experimental diabetic cardiomyopathy are ameliorated by alpha-lipoic acid. *Cardiovasc. Diabetol.* 11, 73-83.

Livak, K. J. & Schmittgen, T. D. (2001). Analysis of relative gene expression data using real-time quantitative PCR and the 2(-Delta Delta C(T)) method. *Methods* 25, 402-408.

López-Otín, C. & Bond, J. S. (2008). Proteases: Multifunctional enzymes in life and disease. *J. Biol. Chem.* 283, 30433-30437.

Loria, P., Lonardo, A. & Anania, F. (2013) Liver and diabetes. A vicious circle. *Hepatol. Res.* 43, 51-64.

Lu, C., He, J. C., Cai, W., Liu, H., Zhu, L. & Vlassara, H. (2004). Advanced glycation endproduct (AGE) receptor 1 is a negative regulator of the inflammatory response to AGE in mesangial cells. *Proc. Natl. Acad. Sci.* USA 101, 11767–11772.

Lu, L., Zhang, Q., Pu, L. J., Peng, W. H., Yan, X. X., Wang, L. J., Chen, Q. J., Zhu, Z. B., Michel, J. B. & Shen, W. (2008). Dysregulation of matrix metalloproteinases and their tissue inhibitors is related to abnormality of left ventricular geometry and function in streptozotocin-induced diabetic minipigs. *Int. J. Exp. Pathol.* 89, 125-137.

Lubec, G., Leban, J., Peyroux, J., Sternberg, M., Pollak, A., Latzka, U. & Coradello, H. (1982). Reduced collagenolytic activity of rat kidneys with steptozotocin diabetes. *Nephron* 30, 357-360.

Martinez, N., Sosa, M., Higa, R., Fornes, D., Capobianco, E. & Jawerbaum, A. (2012). Dietary treatments enriched in olive and safflower oils regulate seric and placental matrix metalloproteinases in maternal diabetes. *Placenta* 33, 8-16.

McLennan, S. V., Kelly, D. J., Cox, A. J., Cao, Z., Lyons, J. G., Yue, D. K. & Gilbert, R. E. (2002). Decreased matrix degradation in diabetic nephropathy: effects of ACE inhibition on the expression and activities of matrix metalloproteinases. *Diabetologia* 45, 268-275.

McLennan, S. V., Kelly, D. J., Schache, M., Waltham, M., Dy, V., Langham, R. G., Yue, D. K. & Gilbert, R. E. (2007). Advanced glycation end products decrease mesangial cell MMP-7: a role in matrix accumulation in diabetic nephropathy? *Kidney Int.* 72, 481-488.

McLennan, S. V., Yue, D. K. & Turtle, J. R. (1998). Effect of glucose on matrix metalloproteinase activity in mesangial cells. *Nephron* 79, 293–298.

Mohanam, S. & Bose, S. M. (1983). Influence of streptozotocin- and alloxan-induced diabetes in the rat on collagenase and certain lysosomal enzymes in relation to the degradation of connective tissue proteins. *Diabetologia* 25, 66-70.

Nakamura, T., Fukui, M., Ebihara, I., Osada, S., Tomino, Y. & Koide, H. (1994). Abnormal gene expression of matrix metalloproteinases and their inhibitor in glomeruli from diabetic rats. *Ren. Physiol, Biochem.* 17, 316-325.

Oltman, C. L., Davidson, E. P., Coppey, L. J., Kleinschmidt, T. L., Dake, B. & Yorek, M. A. (2011). Role of the effect of inhibition of neutral endopeptidase on vascular and neural complications in streptozotocin-induced diabetic rats. *Eur. J. Pharmacol.* 650, 556-562.

Peres, G. B., Juliano, M. A., Aguiar, J. A. K. & Michelacci, Y. M. (2013b). Streptozotocin-induced diabetes mellitus affects lysosomal enzymes in rat liver. *Braz. J. Med. Biol. Res.* (submitted).

Peres, G. B., Juliano, M. A., Simoes, M. J. & Michelacci, Y. M. (2013a) Lysosomal enzymes are decreased in the kidney of diabetic rats. *Biochim. Biophys. Acta.* 1832, 85-95.

Pustovrh, C., Jawerbaum, A., Sinner, D., White, V., Capobianco, E. & González, E. (2002). Metalloproteinase 2 activity and modulation in uterus from neonatal streptozotocin-induced diabetic rats during embryo implantation. *Reprod. Fertil. Dev.* 14, 479-485.

Pustovrh, M. C., Capobianco, E., Martínez, N., Higa, R., White, V. & Jawerbaum, A. (2009). MMP/ TIMP balance is modulated in vitro by 15dPGJ(2) in fetuses and placentas from diabetic rats. *Eur. J. Clin. Invest.* 39, 1082-1190.

Pustovrh, M. C., Jawerbaum, A., Capobianco, E., White, V., López-Costa, J. J. & González, E. (2005). Increased matrix metalloproteinases 2 and 9 in placenta of diabetic rats at midgestation. *Placenta* 26, 339-348.

Reckelhoff, J. F., Tygart, V. L., Mitias, M. M. & Walcott, S. L. (1993). STZ-induced diabetes results in decreased activity of glomerular cathepsin and metalloprotease in rats, *Diabetes* 42, 1425-1432.

Schaefer, L., Schaefer, R. M., Ling, H., Teschner, M. & Heidland, A. (1994). Renal proteinases and kidney hypertrophy in experimental diabetes. *Diabetologia* 37, 567-571.

Schalkwijk, C. G. & Stehouwer, C. D. (2005). Vascular complications in diabetes mellitus: the role of endothelial dysfunction. *Clin. Sci.* 109, 143–159.

Schmidt, A. M., Yan, S. D., Wautier, J. L. & Stern, D. (1999). Activation of receptor for advanced glycation end products: a mechanism for chronic vascular dysfunction in diabetic vasculopathy and atherosclerosis. *Circ. Res.* 19, 489–497.

Severson, D. L. (2004). Diabetic cardiomyopathy: recent evidence from mouse models of type 1 and type 2 diabetes. *Can. J. Physiol. Pharmacol.* 82, 813–823.

Shapiro, S. D., Kelley, D. & Kobayashi, D. (2001). Measurement of metalloproteinase. *Methods in Mol. Med.* 56, 383-390.

Shechter, P., Boner, G. & Rabkin, R. (1994). Tubular cell protein degradation in early diabetic renal hypertrophy. *J. Am. Soc. Nephrol.* 4, 1582-1587.

Singh, R., Song, R. H., Alavi, N., Pegoraro, A. A., Singh, A. K. & Leehey, D. J. (2001). High glucose decreases matrix metalloproteinase-2 activity in rat mesangial cells via transforming growth factor-beta1. *Exp. Nephrol.* 9, 249-257.

Sinha-Hikim, I., Shen, R., Nzenwa, I., Gelfand, R., Mahata, S. K., Sinha-Hikim, A. P. (2011). Minocycline suppresses oxidative stress and attenuates fetal cardiac myocyte apoptosis triggered by in utero cocaine exposure. *Apoptosis* 16, 563-573.

Song, R. H., Singh, A. K. & Leehey, D. J. (1999). Decreased glomerular proteinase activity in the streptozotocin diabetic rat. *Am. J. Nephrol.* 19, 441-446.

Soro-Paavonen, A., Watson, A. M., Li, J., Paavonen, K., Koitka, A., Calkin, A. C., Barit, D., Coughlan, M. T., Drew, B. G., Lancaster, G. I., Thomas, M., Forbes, J. M., Nawroth,

P. P., Bierhaus, A., Cooper, M. E. & Jandeleit-Dahm, K. A. (2008). Receptor for advanced glycation end products (RAGE) deficiency attenuates the development of atherosclerosis in diabetes. *Diabetes* 57, 2461-2469.

Spinale, F. G. (2013). Epilysin (matrix metalloproteinase-28) joins the matrix metalloproteinase team on the field of postmyocardial infarction remodeling. *Circ. Res.* 112, 579-582.

Sun, S., Wang, Y., Li, Q., Tian, Y. J., Liu, M. H. & Yu, Y. H. (2006). Effects of benazepril on renal function and kidney expression of matrix metalloproteinase-2 and tissue inhibitor of metalloproteinase-2 in diabetic rats. *Chin. Med. J.* 119, 814-821.

Sung, P. H., Sun, C. K., Ko, S. F., Chang, L. T., Sheu, J. J., Lee, F. Y., Wu, C. J., Chua, S. & Yip, H. K. (2009). Impact of hyperglycemic control on left ventricular myocardium. A molecular and cellular basic study in a diabetic rat model. *Int. Heart J.* 50, 191-206.

Takahashi, N. & Takasu, S. (2011). A close relationship between type 1 diabetes and vitamin A-deficiency and matrix metalloproteinase and hyaluronidase activities in skin tissues. *Exp. Dermatol.* 20, 899-904.

Tamarat, R., Silvestre, J. S., Huijberts, M., Benessiano, J., Ebrahimian, T. G., Duriez, M., Wautier, M. P., Wautier, J. L. & Lévy, B. I. (2003). Blockade of advanced glycation end-product formation restores ischemia-induced angiogenesis in diabetic mice. *Proc. Natl. Acad. Sci.* USA 100, 8555-8560.

The Diabetes Control and Complications Trial Research Group (1993). The effect of intensive treatment of diabetes on the development and progression of long-term complications in insulin-dependent diabetes mellitus. *N. Engl. J. Med.* 329, 977–986.

Thornalley, P. J. (2005). Dicarbonyl intermediates in the maillard reaction. *Ann. N. Y. Acad. Sci.* 1043, 111–117.

Torffvit, O. (2003). Hyperglycaemia in diabetes: impact on nephropathy and cardiac risk. *Nephrol. Dial. Transplant.* 18, 1711-1715.

Uemura, S., Matsushita, H., Li, W., Glassford, A. J., Asagami, T., Lee, K. H., Harrison, D. G. & Tsao, P. S. (2001). Diabetes mellitus enhances vascular matrix metalloproteinase activity: role of oxidative stress. *Circ. Res.* 88, 1291-1298.

UK Prospective Diabetes Study (UKPDS) Group (1998). Intensive blood-glucose control with sulphonylureas or insulin compared with conventional treatment and risk of complications in patients with type 2 diabetes (UKPDS 33). *Lancet* 352, 837– 853.

Vadla, G. P. & Vellaichamy, E. (2012). Anti-fibrotic cardio protective efficacy of aminoguanidine against streptozotocin induced cardiac fibrosis and high glucose induced collagen up regulation in cardiac fibroblasts. *Chem. Biol. Interact.* 197, 119-128.

Van Linthout, S., Seeland, U., Riad, A., Eckhardt, O., Hohl, M., Dhayat, N., Richter, U., Fischer, J. W., Böhm, M., Pauschinger, M., Schultheiss, H. P. & Tschöpe, C. (2008). Reduced MMP-2 activity contributes to cardiac fibrosis in experimental diabetic cardiomyopathy. *Basic Res. Cardiol.* 103, 319-327.

Varani, J., Perone, P., Merfert, M. G., Moon, S. E., Larkin, D. & Stevens, M. J. (2002). All-trans retinoic acid improves structure and function of diabetic rat skin in organ culture. *Diabetes* 51, 3510-3516.

Vlassara, H., Fuh, H., Makita, Z., Krungkrai, S., Cerami, A. & Bucala, R. (1992). Exogenous advanced glycosylation end products induce complex vascular dysfunction in normal animals: a model for diabetic and aging complications. *Proc. Natl. Acad. Sci.* USA 89, 12043–12047.

Vu, T. H. & Werb, Z. (2000). Matrix metalloproteinases: effectors of development and normal physiology. *Genes Dev.* 14, 2123-2133.

Williams, J. M., Zhang, J., North, P., Lacy, S., Yakes, M., Dahly-Vernon, A. & Roman, R. J. (2011). Evaluation of metalloprotease inhibitors on hypertension and diabetic nephropathy. *Am. J. Physiol. Renal Physiol.* 300, F983-F998.

Wu, K., Setty, S., Mauer, S. M., Killen, P., Nagase, H., Michael, A. F. & Tsilibary, E. C. (1997). Altered kidney matrix gene expression in early stages of experimental diabetes. *Acta Anat.* (Basel) 158, 155-165.

Xie, X. Y., Yang, C., Ren, M., Hao, S. Y., Zhu, P. & Yan, L. (2012). Inhibition of matrix metalloproteinase 9 expression in rat dermal fibroblasts using small interfering RNA. *J. Am. Podiatr. Med. Assoc.* 102, 299-308.

Yan, S. F., Ramasamy, R. & Schmidt, A. M. (2010). The RAGE axis: a fundamental mechanism signaling danger to the vulnerable vasculature. *Circ. Res.* 106, 842–853.

Yan, S. F., Ramasamy, R., Naka, Y. & Schmidt, A. M. (2003). Glycation, inflammation, and RAGE: a scaffold for the macrovascular complications of diabetes and beyond. *Circ. Res.* 93, 1159-1169.

Yang, C., Zhu, P., Yan, L., Chen, L., Meng, R. & Lao, G. (2009). Dynamic changes in matrix metalloproteinase 9 and tissue inhibitor of metalloproteinase 1 levels during wound healing in diabetic rats. *J. Am. Podiatr. Med. Assoc.* 99, 489-496.

Zhang, F., Banker, G., Liu, X., Suwanabol, P. A., Lengfeld, J., Yamanouchi, D., Kent, K. C. & Liu, B. (2011). The novel function of advanced glycation end products in regulation of MMP-9 production. *J. Surg. Res.* 171, 871-876.

Zhao, Z., Huang, G., Wang, B. & Zhong, Y. (2013). Inhibition of NF-kappaB activation by Pyrrolidine dithiocarbamate partially attenuates hippocampal MMP-9 activation and improves cognitive deficits in streptozotocin-induced diabetic rats. *Behav. Brain. Res.* 238, 44-47.

In: Streptozotocin: Uses, Mechanism of Action and Side Effects ISBN: 978-1-63117-255-7
Editor: Elizabeth L. Gauthier 

*Chapter 6*

# GENOTOXIC EFFECTS OF STREPTOZOTOCIN

***Alejandro D. Bolzán****

Laboratorio de Citogenética y Mutagénesis, Instituto Multidisciplinario de Biología Celular (IMBICE, CCT-CONICET La Plata-CICPBA), La Plata, Argentina

## ABSTRACT

Streptozotocin (Streptozocin, STZ, CAS No. 18883-66-4) is a monofunctional nitrosourea derivative isolated from *Streptomyces achromogenes* with broad spectrum antibiotic activity and antineoplastic properties. This compound is often used to induce diabetes *mellitus* in experimental animals through its toxic effects on pancreatic β-cells. STZ is a potent alkylating agent known to directly methylate DNA, thus inducing DNA damage by alkylation of specific sites on DNA bases. DNA lesions produced by STZ includes double and single-strand breaks, covalent adducts and alkali-labile sites. Moreover, STZ induces unscheduled DNA synthesis and DNA synthesis inhibition. Severe DNA damage by STZ results in cell death by apoptosis or necrosis. The DNA strand breaks resulting from the alkylating action of STZ can lead to chromosomal rearrangements. Accordingly, STZ tests positive in the chromosomal aberrations, micronuclei and sister chromatid exchanges assays. In addition, this antibiotic was found to be mutagenic in bacterial assays and eukaryotic cells and is also carcinogenic: a single administration of STZ induces tumors in rat kidney, liver, and pancreas. Since STZ is used as an antineoplastic agent for the treatment of pancreatic neuroendocrine carcinomas, the study of its genotoxicity is of great importance to understand the genomic instability associated with chemotherapy regimens involving administration of this antibiotic. Therefore, the purpose of this chapter is to summarize the current knowledge regarding the genotoxic effects of STZ.

* Corresponding author: Tel: 54-0221-4210112, Fax: 54-0221-4253320; E-mail: abolzan@imbice.org.ar / abolzan@imbice.gov.ar.

# 1. INTRODUCTION

Streptozotocin (Streptozocin, STZ, Zanosar®, CAS No. 18883-66-4) is a monofunctional nitrosourea derivative that was first isolated from the bacterium *Streptomyces achromogenes* fermentation broth [1]. Its molecular structure has been described elsewhere [2] and corresponds to a 2-deoxy-d-glucose molecule substituted at $C_2$ with an *N*-methyl-*N*-nitrosourea group (Figure 1). The systematic (IUPAC) name of STZ is (2-deoxy-2-({[methyl(nitroso)amino]carbonyl}amino)-β-D-glucopyranose).

STZ has broad spectrum antibiotic activity [1] and is often used to induce experimental Type I diabetes *mellitus* in different species of laboratory animals through its toxic effects on insulin producing pancreatic β-cells [3,4]. STZ toxicity is known to be mediated by poly-ADP-ribose polymerase. STZ is transported to β-cells via the glucose transporter GLUT2 and causes DNA damage leading to increased activity of poly-(ADP-ribose)-polymerase (PARP-1) to repair DNA [5,6]. STZ-induced diabetes has been also reported in Young Non-Obese Diabetic (NOD) mice [7] and cynomolgus monkeys [8,9].

Due to its DNA alkylating properties, STZ belongs to a group of antineoplastic drugs known as alkylnitrosoureas, chemical compounds that are clinically active against a broad range of tumors [10-12]. In particular, STZ has been used in combination with doxorubicin, 5-fluorouracil (FU), cisplatin and/or radiation for the clinical treatment of pancreatic neuroendocrine carcinomas [13-19]. However, treatment failure and disease relapse have been observed in some cases, due to the development of resistance to STZ, a phenomenon usually observed in cells treated with alkylating compounds [20-22]. In effect, some types of cells are highly or even completely resistant to the toxic effects of STZ. For example, Capucci et al., [22] reported that Chinese hamster V79 cells are resistant to the genotoxic effects of STZ, Yan and Wright [23] based on their results on human islet grafts in mice found that human β-cells are exceedingly resistant to STZ, and Fazio and Pin [24] reported that mice lacking Mist1 transcription factor are resistant to STZ-induced β-cell damage.

Despite of its antineoplastic properties, STZ is carcinogenic: a single intravenous or intraperitoneal administration of this antibiotic induces tumors in rat kidney, liver, and pancreas [25-31], lung, kidney, and uterine tumors in mice [30], and liver tumors in hamster [32,33]. STZ also induces neoplastic transformation in primary cultures of human and rat kidney cells [34]. Recently, in a study carried out in diabetic Wistar-Furth rats, it was shown that STZ-induced diabetic rat model is not suitable for long-term studies because this antibiotic causes progressive renal tumorigenesis [31]. The International Agency for Research on Cancer (IARC) indicates that *STZ should be regarded for practical purposes as it were carcinogenic to humans* [35]. For that reason, the IARC Monographs on The Evaluation of Carcinogenic Risks to Humans classifies STZ within Group 2B of agents [*The agent (mixture) is possibly carcinogenic to humans. The exposure circumstance entails exposures that are possibly carcinogenic to humans*] [36].

Besides its antibiotic and diabetogenic properties, STZ is genotoxic in a variety of assays, including microbial mutagenesis, DNA strand breaks, alkali-labile sites, unscheduled DNA synthesis, micronucleus test, chromosomal aberrations (CAs), and sister chromatid exchanges (SCEs) [37]. The purpose of this chapter is to summarize the current knowledge regarding the genotoxic effects of STZ. Thus, in the following sections we will consider in detail each one of them.

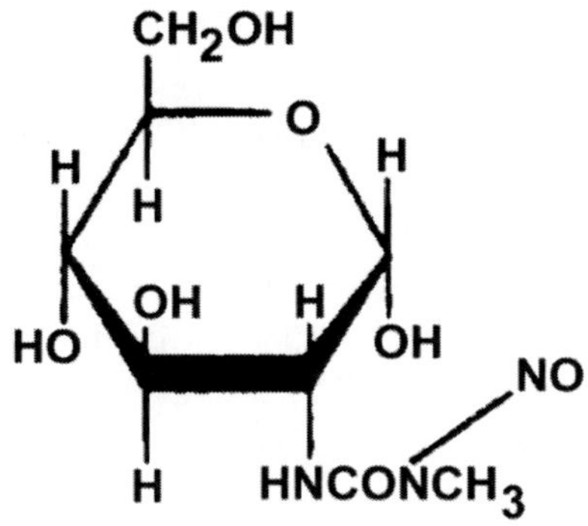


Figure 1. Chemical structure of Streptozotocin (STZ).

## 2. GENOTOXIC EFFECTS OF STZ

### 2.1. Effects of STZ on DNA

As previously indicated, STZ is a potent alkylating agent which directly methylates DNA [38-40]. STZ administration produces significant levels of $N^7$-methylguanine ($N^7$-MeG), $O^6$-methylguanine ($O^6$-MeG), $N^7$-methyladenine, and $N^3$-methyladenine DNA adducts in rat kidney [39]. It was shown that the base adduct of principal biological significance resulting from DNA methylation by STZ is $N^7$-MeG, since more than 70% of DNA methylation occurs at the $N^7$ position of guanine [39,41-44]. A significant fraction of the lesions produced in the DNA by STZ are repaired by the enzyme $O^6$-alkylguanine DNA alkyltransferase, encoded by the gene MGMT [45]. Although the $O^6$-MeG adducts and other less common methylated bases such as $O^4$-and $O^2$-methylthymidine may be more significant promutagenic lesions than $N^7$-MeG [46], the latter may also be mutagenic, since apurinic sites are promutagenic due to preferential incorporation of adenine by DNA polymerases at abasic sites [47]. For this reason, $N^7$-MeG is considered a good indicator of overall DNA damage by STZ.

In addition to covalent adducts, STZ induces single and double DNA strand breaks and alkali-labile sites. It was shown that STZ induces DNA strand breaks and alkali-labile sites in Chinese hamster V79 cells [48] and rat liver [49], DNA strand breaks in kidney and liver of rats [50] and in rat pancreatic islets [51-53], and DNA strand breaks and $N^7$-MeG adducts in neonatal rat β cells [54]. Moreover, STZ induces DNA strand breaks and mutations in the liver and kidney of male C57BL/6 mice dosed i.p., as determined by a microgel electrophoresis assay and the Lacl transgenic mouse mutation assay, respectively, at levels of 25–150 mg/kg [55]. Imaeda et al., [56] investigated the effects of STZ on DNA damage in the liver and kidney of mice by using the alkaline (pH>13) single-cell gel electrophoresis assay (comet assay). A single i.p. injection of STZ (150 mg/kg) caused DNA damage in the liver and kidney, which recovered slowly with time. Likewise, using the alkaline comet assay, Blasiak et al. [57] showed that STZ (0.01-100 μM) induced DNA damage in normal human lymphocytes and HeLa cancer cells in a concentration-dependent manner. Lymphocytes were able to remove the induced DNA damage within 30-min repair incubation, whereas HeLa cells completed the repair in 60 min. Moreover, by applying the alkaline *in vivo* comet assay, Nesslany et al. [58] showed that STZ (20 mg/kg) induced DNA damage in isolated kidney cells from Sprague-Dawley male rats. Induction of DNA damage by STZ was also studied in different organs of Sprague Dawley rats by Kushwaha et al. [59] using the alkaline and the endonuclease-III (Endo III) and formamidopyrimidine-DNA glycosylase (FPG) modified comet assays. STZ induced oxidative DNA damage in all tested tissues (lung, liver, heart, aorta, kidney, pancreas and peripheral blood lymphocytes). More recently, Lima et al. [60] evaluated the genotoxicity of STZ (in terms of DNA damage) in lymphocytes from pregnant Wistar rats with severe or mild diabetes and in whole blood samples from their newborns. The oxidative DNA damage induced by STZ was evaluated by applying the Endo III and FPG modified comet assays in blood samples from rats sacrificed at day 21 of pregnancy. The rats with mild diabetes and their offspring showed higher FPG-sensitive sites (reflecting damage induced by hyperglycemia), whereas the rats with severe diabetes and their offspring showed higher FPG and Endo III-sensitive sites (reflecting oxidative DNA damage) [60].

Induction and repair of DNA strand breaks and alkali-labile sites by STZ was investigated by several research groups. For example, Mossman et al. [61] showed that DNA single-strand breaks induced by STZ in a rat insulinoma cell line (RINr 38) can be repaired in a time-dependent manner, with most repair completed by 24 h after exposure to the antibiotic. Using the same cell line, Pettepher et al. [62] demonstrated that STZ induces alkali-labile sites in a dose-dependent manner within the mitochondrial DNA and that these lesions can also be repaired. In effect, 8 h after exposure to STZ, 55% of the lesions induced in the mitochondrial DNA were removed. The level of repair of mitochondrial DNA damage increased to 70 % after 24 h of exposure to the antibiotic, but only 46% of $N^7$-MeG adducts produced across the entire genome were removed. In addition, Fram et al. [63] found that STZ caused single-stranded DNA breaks in *Escherichia coli* strains not proficient in recombinational repair lacking either RecA protein or *RecBC* gene products. DNA breaks in RecBC cells were repaired, but those present in RecA cells were not. These findings point out the critical importance of recombinational repair in amending the DNA damage caused by STZ in *E. coli*. Kraynak et al. [64] analyzed the extent and persistence of STZ-induced DNA damage and cell proliferation in the kidney of male Sprague-Dawley rats (given intravenous injections of 0.25 to 60 mg/kg STZ) using and *in vivo* alkaline elution assay for DNA strand breaks and a BrdUrd labeling assay for cell replication, providing evidence that the cellular and molecular repair responses to a single diabetogenic dose of this compound are prolonged, requiring up to 3 weeks to complete. A dose of 2.5 mg/kg STZ was the lowest one to induce detectable DNA strand breaks and extensive damage was produced by the diabetogenic dose of 60 mg/kg. Significant DNA damage was detected up to 14 days, with return to near background levels by 20 days after STZ treatment. Treatment with 60 mg/kg STZ was associated with increases in BrdUrd labeling indices 4 and 9 days after treatment, with resolution by 27 days [64].

Another genotoxic effect of STZ is the induction of unscheduled DNA synthesis (UDS). This effect has been observed by Tyson and Mirsalis in isolated rat kidney cells following *in vivo* treatment of male Fisher-344 rats with STZ [65] and confirmed by Shepherd et al. [66] using cultured normal rat pancreatic epithelial cells. In the latter case, the concentration of STZ that caused 50% inhibition in colony formation (LD50) was 2 mM. Induction of DNA damage by STZ was also evident by an increased expression of growth arrest and DNA damage-inducible genes *gadd* 153 and *gadd* 45 observed in rat pancreatic islets treated with the antibiotic [67]. More recently, using DNA microarray technology, Kume et al. [68,69] found that STZ induces changes in gene expression in mouse liver (STZ dose of 200 mg/kg)

[68] and primary cultured hepatocytes (STZ concentrations of 1-100 mM) [69]. Results were similar in both *in vivo* and *in vitro* systems: some genes were up-regulated by STZ (cell cycle/apoptosis related genes, immune/allergy related genes, and stress response/xenobiotic metabolism related genes), while others (genes related to glucose, lipid and protein metabolism) were down-regulated by STZ. These results strongly support the hypothesis that many of the hepatic alterations including histopathological and gene expression changes observed in STZ-treated animals are induced by a direct effect of the antibiotic. On the other hand, studies in DNA repair-deficient *E. coli* mutants have shown that STZ inhibits DNA synthesis [63]. This effect was demonstrated in strains not proficient in recombinational repair (which lack either RecA protein or *RecBC* gene products) and in *E. coli* cells lacking both 3-methyladenine DNA glycosylases I (tag) and II (alkA). DNA synthesis inhibition was also demonstrated in Chinese hamster cells CHO-9 and V79 [44].

Besides the above mentioned effects on the DNA molecule, STZ was shown to induce cell death by apoptosis and necrosis. Cell death by apoptosis induced by STZ treatment was observed in rat pancreatic β cell lines HIT-T15 and RINm5F [70]. In addition, STZ at low doses induced cell death by apoptosis and at high doses caused cell death by necrosis in the murine pancreatic-cell line INS-1 [71]. Higher rates of apoptosis, as compared to necrosis, were observed when cells were exposed to 15 mM STZ for 1 h followed by a 24 h recovery period. Higher doses of STZ (30 mM) caused the cells to undergo necrosis (22%) as well as apoptosis (17%). Moreover, Harel et al. [72] found that the immortal human keratinocyte HaCat cell line treated with 10 and 20 mM STZ showed a significant increase in apoptosis (3.9 and 6.7-fold, respectively), but not in necrosis, compared to naive cells. Moreover, STZ was shown to produce apoptosis in rat INS-1 cells via activation of caspase-3, a proteolytic enzyme which plays a central role at end-stage apoptosis [73].

On the other hand, though STZ *per se* does not induce DNA inter-strand cross-links, studies in human cell lines of the $Mer^+$ phenotype (i.e. proficient in the repair of guanine $O^6$ alkylations) showed that this antibiotic apparently saturates the monoadduct repair system and allows other alkylating drugs to form these lesions in the DNA molecule [74,75].

## 2.2. Mechanism of Induction of DNA Damage by STZ. The Role of Free Radicals

The mechanism of induction of DNA damage by STZ was investigated more than a decade ago by Murata et al. [76], using a human cell line and $^{32}P$-labeled DNA fragments isolated from human genes. It was found that STZ frequently initiates DNA modification at guanines, especially at the middle guanine in runs of three and at the guanine at the 3'-end of runs of two guanines. Sodium acetate and sodium chloride (both of which can reduce the reactivity of methylating agents to DNA via the sodium cation) inhibited the induction of DNA damage by STZ, but scavengers for reactive oxygen species and nitric oxide (NO) were ineffective in doing so [76]. These findings suggest that STZ induces DNA damage by methylation of guanines via methyl cations. Although it is generally accepted that the cytotoxicity produced by STZ depends on DNA alkylation [38,39], several lines of evidence indicate that free radicals are also involved in the production of DNA damage and cytotoxicity by STZ. Thus, for example, it was found that STZ enhances $O_2^-$ radical generation by the xanthine oxidase system of pancreatic cells [77,78] and stimulates $H_2O_2$

generation, causing DNA fragmentation in isolated rat pancreatic islets [79]. The latter effects were evident at a concentration of 0.1 mM and were maximal at 1 mM of STZ. Moreover, it was shown that STZ generates $OH^{-}$ radicals in diabetic rats [80] and induces DNA double-strand breaks (STZ 0.55 mM for 30 min before culture) in rat pancreatic islet cells [81] which can be prevented by *N*-monomethyl-arginine (which inhibits the inducible form of nitric oxide synthtase) or by nicotinamide (a free radical scavenger). Additional evidence indicates that nitric oxide (NO) is also involved in the production of DNA damage by STZ. In effect, Kroncke et al. [82] demonstrated that NO generation during cellular metabolization of STZ contributes to rat pancreatic islet cell DNA damage. Early DNA-strand breaks induced either by STZ or by the NO donor nitroprusside were both significantly reduced in the presence of an intracellular NO scavenger. Moreover, Chen et al. [83] using transgenic mice found that the overexpression of metallothionein (an inducible cysteine-rich protein with antioxidant properties) in pancreatic β-cells decreases the STZ-induced DNA breakage and cell death. Furthermore, several studies developed about 30 years ago showed that a variety of free radical scavengers, including superoxide dismutase (SOD) [84,85], the artificial SOD, copper(II) (3,5-diisopropylsalicylate)2 [86] the hydroxyl radical scavenger dimethylurea [87], and Vitamin E [88], were found to protect laboratory rats from the diabetogenic effects of STZ. In recent years, several reports have shown the protective effects of a number of compounds against STZ-induced genotoxic effects, providing new evidence concerning the involvement of free radicals and antioxidant enzymes in STZ toxicity. Thus, for example, Imaeda et al. [56] investigated the protective effect of antioxidants on DNA damage induced by STZ (150 mg/kg) in mice liver and kidney, and found that the antioxidants ascorbic acid, trolox, and probucol prevented the increase of DNA damage induced by the antibiotic in these organs. In a similar study [89], these authors showed that fluvastatin, a 3-hydroxy-3-methylglutaryl coenzyme A reductase inhibitor, and its metabolites prevented STZ-induced DNA damage in mice, demonstrating the antioxidative and protective effects of these agents against the genotoxic effect of STZ. Using the alkaline comet assay, Blasiak et al. [57] showed that the DNA damage-inducing effect of STZ (50μM) in normal human lymphocytes and HeLa cancer cells was significantly inhibited by several free radical scavengers, including vitamins E and C (added to the cell cultures at the concentrations of 10 and 50μM), providing additional evidence that free radicals are involved in the genotoxicity of this antibiotic. Very recently, Wayhs et al. [90] analyzed DNA damage in leukocytes from STZ-induced diabetic rats subjected to the forced swimming test, and found that insulin plus clonazepam (a benzodiazepine drug having anxiolytic, anticonvulsant, muscle relaxant, sedative, and hypnotic properties) can protect stressed diabetic rats against DNA damage. Significant reduction in the DNA damage index was observed in diabetic animals treated with insulin, clonazepam, or both agents.

Despite all the above data, there are a few reports suggesting that free radicals may not be involved in the DNA damage by STZ. In effect, it has been reported that exogenous SOD or catalase (CAT) does not prevent the DNA breaks induced by STZ [51-53]. Moreover, in 1999, Murata et al. [76] found that scavengers for reactive oxygen species or NO did not inhibit the induction of DNA damage by STZ in a human cell line. On the other hand, damage induction was inhibited by sodium acetate and sodium chloride, which can reduce the reactivity of methylating agents to DNA via the sodium cation. The reasons for the above disagreements are not clear. They may result from the different experimental approaches employed. Nevertheless, most of the studies performed so far regarding the effect of free radical scavengers on the DNA damage and cytotoxicity induced by STZ clearly support the idea that the genotoxic action of this antibiotic is mediated by free radicals.

In summary, current knowledge about the genotoxic effects of STZ indicates that this compound induces DNA damage by alkylation of specific sites on DNA bases (forming adducts at their N- and O-atoms) and that free radicals (oxidative stress) generated during STZ metabolization seems to play a significant role in the mechanism of DNA damage and cytotoxicity by STZ. DNA lesions produced by STZ includes double and single-strand breaks, covalent adducts and alkali-labile sites. Moreover, STZ is able to induce unscheduled DNA synthesis and also to inhibit DNA synthesis. Severe DNA damage by STZ results in cell death by apoptosis or necrosis. Furthermore, as we will see in the next section of this chapter, DNA strand breaks resulting from the alkylating action of STZ can lead to chromosomal rearrangements.

## 2.3. Effects of STZ on Chromosomes

The first reports on the clastogenic effects of STZ in mammalian cells were published more than four decades ago [91,92]. These studies showed that STZ inhibits progress of cell into mitosis (the drug-induced block occurring in G2) and cell proliferation, and that this antibiotic induces CAs, mostly of chromatid-type, like breaks, gaps and exchanges. However, it was not until the last two decades that the chromosomal effects of this antibiotic began to be intensively investigated. Using the classical CAs assay, several investigators found that STZ produces all types of aberrations in the first post-treatment mitosis (i.e. dicentrics, rings, deletions, exchanges, breaks and gaps) but with a clear predominance of chromatid-type aberrations in all of the systems studied. These systems included Chinese hamster cells, mosquito cells and human lymphocytes [22,93-96]. In particular, it was found that STZ (1 mM for 1 h at 37°C) induces CAs (mainly chromatid-type) in cycling but not in unstimulated human lymphocytes, indicating that this antibiotic does not induce CAs in the G0 phase of the cell cycle [96]. However, no induction of CAs by STZ in isolated lymphocytes was detected, probably because of a lethal or cytotoxic effect of this compound, as suggested by the marked depression of the mitotic index observed in some samples and the absence of metaphase cells in some chromosome preparations [96]. A similar effect was previously observed in mouse leukemia L1210 cells [91,97].

It has been shown that agents that induce CAs mainly because of the formation of $O^6$-MeG adducts will give a much larger increase in aberrations in the second than in the first metaphases after treatment [22,98,99], and that *N*-alkylations are the major source of aberrations observed in the first post-treatment mitosis [100]. The abovementioned study in human lymphocytes suggests that STZ does not exhibit a delayed clastogenic effect, at least in these cells, since no induction of CAs was found in second division metaphases from 72 h cultures [96]. However, it was found that under similar experimental conditions to those previously used with peripheral blood lymphocytes, STZ produces a concentration-dependent increase in the frequency of CAs and induces severe chromosome damage (fragmentation and pulverization) in COLO320DM and HSR cell lines (derived from a human neuroendocrine colon carcinoma) *in vitro* [101]. Fragmentation and pulverization of COLO320DM and HSR chromosomes were observed in cells that had progressed beyond the first metaphase after treatment, and a higher percentage of metaphases with pulverized chromosomes were found in cells after the second than after the first mitosis after STZ treatment. These findings suggest that STZ has a persistent and delayed clastogenic effect on human COLO320 cells. Overall, the above studies show that the chromosomal sensitivity of human cells to STZ depends on the cell type.

The effects of STZ on chromosomes were also studied using the micronucleus and sister-chromatid exchanges (SCEs) assays. This antibiotic was found to be a good inducer of micronuclei in mouse bone marrow cells [102,103] and SCEs in mammalian and insect cells [22,93,95,96,104]. Liegibel et al. [102] found that STZ is active in the mouse bone marrow micronucleus assay following a single intraperitoneal injection of 150-180 mg/kg. A few years ago, Vikram et al. [105] analyzed the genotoxic potential of STZ (10, 30 and 100 mg/kg x 1, 3 and 7 days) in rat peripheral blood reticulocytes and bone marrow polychromatic erythrocytes using the micronucleus test. They found that STZ induced micronucleus in a dose-dependent manner in both neonatal and young rat peripheral blood reticulocytes as well as in bone marrow polychromatic erythrocytes. However, significant induction of micronucleus in adult rats was only observed in bone marrow polychromatic erythrocytes. In addition, using the comet assay in bone marrow cells and peripheral blood lymphocytes of young rats, these authors found that STZ (30 mg/kg x 3 days) induces significant DNA damage. Thus, it seems that neonatal and young rats are more suitable over adult rats for the peripheral blood micronucleus assay to test the genotoxicity of STZ. It has been shown that the clastogenicity of STZ in mouse bone marrow, as measured by the micronucleus assay, can be potentiated by prior treatment with the $O^6$-alkylguanine-DNA-alkyltransferase inactivator $O^6$-benzylguanine [103]. This effect was found to be significantly inhibited in myeloablated mice reconstituted with bone marrow expressing the $O^6$-benzylguanine-resistant mutant of human $O^6$-alkylguanine-DNA-alkyltransferase (hATPA/GA) as a result of retroviral gene transfer [103]. This finding indicates that $O^6$-MeG adducts are clastogenic *in vivo* and establishes the enzyme $O^6$-alkylguanine-DNA-alkyltransferase as a major protective mechanism against such DNA damage.

Induction of SCEs and CAs in different Chinese hamster cell lines were analyzed by Capucci et al. [22,93]. They found that STZ induces SCEs and CAs in CHO-9 cells and its mutant EM-C11 cell line (hypersensitive to alkylating agents), although the latter was found to be more sensitive than parental cells to the killing and CAs-inducing effects of the antibiotic [93]. Moreover, V79 cells were found to be more resistant than CHO-9 cells to the induction of SCEs and CAs by the antibiotic [22]. Human lymphocytes were found to be highly sensitive to the induction of SCEs by STZ [96]. STZ was found to produce a similar effect on the frequency of SCEs in lymphocytes obtained from whole blood cultures and purified lymphocytes, suggesting that blood components do not interfere in the SCEs response of these cells. Like S-dependent agents, STZ was found to induce SCEs at concentrations lower than those required for the induction of CAs [96].

STZ clastogenic effects have been recently investigated using the Fluorescence *in situ* hybridization (FISH) technique with a peptide nucleic acid (PNA) telomeric probe [106,107], in order to analyze the induction of CAs involving telomeres and interstitial telomeric sequences by this compound. It was found that STZ induces the formation of incomplete chromosome elements (i.e., lacking one or both chromosome ends) in Chinese hamster embryo cells (i.e., CHE cell line), and that chromosomal incompleteness, in the form of incomplete chromosomes (lacking one end) and terminal fragments (i.e., acentric fragments exhibiting telomeric signals at only one end) is a very common event following exposure to

STZ. In effect, about 40% metaphases present in cell cultures treated with the antibiotic contained one or more pairs of incomplete chromosome elements [106]. Moreover, centric (incomplete chromosomes) and acentric (terminal fragments) incomplete chromosome elements were the only unstable chromosome-type aberrations induced by STZ in CHE cells, which suggests that all of the excess acentric fragments (i.e., excess of fragments resulting from the formation of dicentric and ring chromosomes) induced by STZ originate from terminal deletions [106]. In addition, STZ showed curvilinear concentration–response curves for induction of incomplete chromosome elements and terminal fragments, suggesting that incomplete chromosome elements are formed by a mechanism involving two-hit events, i.e., these aberrations are caused by the interaction of two STZ-induced DNA lesions (probably DNA double-strand breaks) [106]. No further studies on the effects of STZ on telomeres have been reported so far. Concerning the effects of STZ on interstitial telomeric sequences (i.e., those ones located at the centromeric region or between the centromere and the telomere of chromosomes), it was found that in Chinese hamster ovary (CHO) cells this compound induces CAs involving these sequences, but the chromosomal regions containing these repeats are not the preferential target of the clastogenic action of STZ [107]. CHO cells were exposed to increasing concentrations of STZ, and CAs were analyzed in the first mitosis after treatment. The frequency of CAs directly involving interstitial telomeric sequences increased in STZ-treated cells by a factor of 2.6 (2 mM) and 3.6 (4 mM) when compared with the frequency of these aberrations in control cells. However, no significant differences were found between control and exposed cells in the percentage of aberrations directly involving ITSs, demonstrating that these repeat regions are not preferentially involved in the chromosome damage induced by STZ. In addition, STZ did not alter telomerase activity, suggesting that this enzyme may not be involved in the induction of CAs by this compound [107].

Despite the clastogenic capacity of STZ, it has been demonstrated that there are mammalian cells, including human cancer cells, which are highly or even completely resistant to the clastogenic and SCEs-inducing effect of STZ and other methylating compounds [21,22,99,100,104,108-111]. This resistance has been usually ascribed to the activity of the DNA repair protein methylguanine-DNA-methyltransferase (MGMT), which demethylates mainly $O^6$-MeG residues from the DNA molecule [20,21]. In fact, methylating agents like STZ were found to decrease MGMT levels by introducing $O^6$-MeG residues in DNA which are then repaired by the MGMT protein [112-114]. By decreasing MGMT activity, STZ enhances the cytotoxicity of other alkylating compounds [115-116]. Mammalian cells that express a high level of resistance to methylating compounds usually express detectable amounts of MGMT and are defined as $Mer^+$ [108]. Conversely, mammalian cells that do not express MGMT activity are defined as $Mer^-$. Human and rodent cells that do not express MGMT activity and are resistant to methylation have also been reported, suggesting that the cellular resistance of these cells to the cytotoxic effect of DNA methylation may be determined by processes other than MGMT activity [44,109,110,117,118]. Some hypotheses have been proposed to explain the resistance of mammalian $Mer^-$ cells to DNA-alkylation damage. Thus, to explain the resistance of CHO clones to MNU-induced DNA damage, Aquilina et al. [119] suggested the existence of a possible defect or loss in the mismatch repair system of these cells. Alternatively, the resistance of mammalian cells to alkylation damage could be explained by the existence of a post-replication repair system [120]. However, a mismatch repair failure or a post-replication repair system are error-prone mechanisms, leading to an increase in the spontaneous and/or induced mutations, by the persistence of the pre-mutagenic lesion $O^6$-MeG in the DNA [109,121]. Capucci et al. [22] demonstrated that STZ is equally effective in inducing point mutations in the cell lines CHO-9 and V79, which are $Mer^-$, despite of the fact that V79 cells were found to be more resistant than CHO-9 cells to the induction of CAs and SCEs by the antibiotic. This indicates that an unknown error-free mechanism of tolerance to DNA methylation damage by STZ is active in V79 cells.

In summary, cytogenetic damage by STZ can be manifested as CAs, SCEs or micronuclei. All the data available indicates that, like S-dependent agents, STZ is an efficient inducer of SCEs. However, unlike agents with a true S-dependent action, STZ induces both chromosome-and chromatid-type aberrations. Therefore, although it can be considered an S-dependent agent, STZ acts on chromosomes both in an S-dependent and S-independent manner.

## 2.4. Mechanism of Induction of Chromosome Damage by STZ. The Role of Free Radicals

Several reports showed that antioxidant compounds and metal chelators significantly inhibit the clastogenic action of STZ, which strongly supports the idea that free radicals are involved in the induction of chromosome damage by this antibiotic. Thus, for example, the addition of liposome-encapsulated antioxidant enzymes SOD (which converts $O_2^-$ into $H_2O_2$) and CAT (which scavenges $H_2O_2$) and the $OH^-$ radical scavenger mannitol were found to prevent to a great extent the yield of STZ-induced chromosome damage in CHO and mosquito cells [94]. This suggests that DNA damage by STZ partially depends on free radicals production and that the protective effect of SOD, CAT and mannitol is due to the scavenging of $O_2^-$, $H_2O_2$, and $OH^-$ radicals generated by the antibiotic. In another study, it was shown that the metal chelating 1,10-phenanthroline (PNT) (a compound that enters the cell and, by forming a complex with iron, prevents the Fenton reaction from occurring, thus blocking the production of the $OH^-$ radical [122]) inhibits to a great extent the yield of STZ-induced CAs but does not prevent the induction of SCEs in CHO and mosquito cells [95]. This fact strongly suggests that intracellular transition metals are implicated in the induction of CAs but not SCEs by STZ, and that the Fenton reaction ($Fe^{2+}$+ $H_2O_2$ → $OH^*$+ $OH^-$+ $Fe^{3+}$) is partially responsible for the production of CAs by this compound. These observations contrast with the previous ones by Eizirik et al. [123], which showed that PNT does not protect against the diabetogenic effects of STZ, and suggest that intracellular transition metals are implicated in the genotoxic but not in the diabetogenic action of this compound.

The most accepted hypothesis about the induction of CAs and SCEs by methylating agents points out that $O^6$-MeG and *N*-methylated bases-induced damage occurs by mismatch repair, which operates at sites of $O^6$-MeG-T or by depurinations and base excision repair intermediates, respectively, which block DNA replication by inhibiting chain elongation, leading to double strand breaks and exchanges [124]. The evidence available for STZ suggests that the induction of CAs also involves the generation of free radicals by the antibiotic in the presence of transition metal ions.

## 2.5. Mutagenesis

### *2.5.1. Bacterial assays*

Several studies have shown that STZ tests positive in all of the Ames tester strains [102,125-130] and is highly mutagenic. The mutagenicity of STZ was tested in the base-pair substitution *Salmonella typhimurium* mutant hisG46 and the hisG46-bearing uvrB excision-repair-deficient mutants TA100, TA1530, TA1535 and TA1950. It was found that STZ is mutagenic for *S. typhimurium* in the absence of a liver microsomal activation system, showing that this compound does not require enzymatic conversion into mutagenic metabolites [125,127]. Moreover, Zimmer and Bhuyan [128] tested the ability of several nitrosoureas to induce mutation (to histidine independence) in the histidine-requiring auxotroph *S. typhimurium* his G46 and found that STZ was almost equally mutagenic to the other nitrosoureas analyzed, although, on a weight basis, STZ was found to be the most mutagenic of all the compounds tested. STZ was found to induce fewer mutations in TA1530 and TA1950 uvrB excision-repair-deficient strains than in the hisG46 excision-proficient strain, indicating that with this compound excision-repair is also a mutation-prone process [129]. Using the Ames test, Franza et al. [130] analyzed the relative mutagenic activities of several nitrosourea antitumor agents, including STZ, and found that this antibiotic was the most mutagenic of all compounds tested, exhibiting at least a 250-fold increase in activity when compared to that of its chloroethyl analog, chlorozotocin. All the compounds tested, including STZ, exhibited increased mutagenicity after incubation with induced rat liver microsomes [130].

STZ was also found to be mutagenic in *E. coli*, inducing SOS repair and causing premutagenic lesions in mutants deficient in SOS repair or exhibiting aberrant mismatch repair [131,132]. Lengeler [133] characterized two classes of mutants of *E. coli* K12 resistant to STZ: mutants resistant to the highest doses of the antibiotic and conditional resistant mutants which are unable to energize or to synthesize the STZ transport system (enzyme IINag-complex of the phosphoenolpyruvate (PEP)-dependent phosphotransferase system, responsible for the uptake of *N*-acetyl-glucosamine, of d-glucosamine and of STZ) under certain growth conditions but do have the transport activity under other conditions.

### *2.5.2. Mammalian cells*

The mutagenic activity of STZ in mammalian systems was first demonstrated in rats (1 or 10 mg/kg of bodyweight) and in mice (400 µ/g per mouse) more than four decades ago by Gabridge et al. [134]. Afterwards, Bhuyan et al. [135] showed that STZ produces mutations to 8-azaguanine (8-AzG) resistance in V79 Chinese hamster cells, and Schmezer et al. [55] using the LacI transgenic mouse mutation assay, showed that STZ induces mutations in the DNA from liver and kidney of male C57BL/6 mice. In addition, Capucci et al. showed that STZ induces mutations at the HPRT locus (6-thioguanine resistant mutations, $HPRT^{-}$) in Chinese hamster V79 and CHO-9 cells as a function of STZ dose [22,93]. These authors also found that the mutants hypersensitive to alkylating agents (EM-C11 cell line) were more sensitive to the mutagenic effects of STZ than the parental (CHO-9) cell line [93]. However, none of these studies analyzed the STZ-induced HPRT mutants in order to determine whether the induced mutations were point mutations or large deletions.

#### *2.5.3. Other eukaryotes*

To our knowledge, there are only a few reports indicating the mutagenic effects of STZ on other eukaryotes. One is that of Browning [136], who tested the mutagenicity of several chemicals and their metabolites in *Drosophila melanogaster* and found that STZ causes X-linked recessive lethal mutations in this species. Likewise, Rodríguez-Arnaiz and Aranda [137] found that STZ tests positive in the w/w + somatic recombination assay in *D. melanogaster*. Furthermore, two reports recently published on the mutagenic effect of STZ showed that STZ is mutagenic in germ cells of repair efficient females of *Drosophila melanogaster*, and that nucleotide excision repair is involved in the removal of nitrogen ethylation damage [138]. Moreover, measuring the specific activity (revertants/mg) of several mutagens including STZ, Araki et al. [139] compared the sensitivity of new *Escherichia coli* tester strains having the TolC outer membrane transport protein mutation (tolC strain) with *E. coli* strains not carrying this mutation (non-tolC strain), and found that tolC strains were less mutagenic to STZ than those of parent strains.

## CONCLUSION

The studies reviewed in this chapter show that STZ is highly genotoxic, causing DNA and chromosome damage by mechanisms which involve free radicals generated during STZ metabolization. DNA lesions produced by STZ include monoadducts, double and single-strand breaks and alkali-labile sites. Moreover, severe DNA damage by STZ results in cell death by apoptosis or necrosis. At the chromosome level, STZ induces micronuclei, CAs and SCEs. Although CAs are usually produced by alkylating compounds by S-dependent mechanisms, present evidence shows that STZ, unlike agents with a true S-dependent action, induces both chromosome-and chromatid-type aberrations. However, like S-dependent agents, STZ is an efficient inducer of SCEs. Therefore, STZ acts on chromosomes both in an S-dependent and S-independent manner.

As reviewed in this chapter, a large body of evidence supports the involvement of free radicals in the production of DNA and CAs by STZ. However, STZ-induced SCEs probably result from the alkylating action of the antibiotic on the DNA molecule. Furthermore, although both $O^6$-MeG and $N^7$-MeG adducts can be converted to CAs and SCEs, since more than 70% of DNA methylation by STZ occurs at the $N^7$ position of guanine, $N^7$-MeG appears as the predominant clastogenic and recombinogenic lesion for this compound.

As previously mentioned, recent data using the FISH technique with a telomeric probe show that, at chromosome level, STZ induces the formation of incomplete chromosomes and terminal fragments in mammalian cells, and suggest that incomplete chromosome elements are formed by a mechanism involving two-hit events, i.e., these aberrations are caused by the interaction of two STZ-induced DNA lesions (probably DNA double-strand breaks) [106]. Moreover, STZ induces chromosomal aberrations involving interstitial telomeric repeats [107]. Given the pivotal role of telomeres and telomeric sequences in genome stability, more studies will be needed to fully elucidate the effect of STZ on telomeres and interstitial telomeric sequences.

Despite of the abovementioned studies, more research focusing on the clastogenic effects of STZ are needed. In particular, studies employing the FISH technique with chromosome painting probes, combined with the use of other types of FISH probes (telomeric, centromeric, etc.) will provide more detailed information regarding the type, frequency and persistence of CAs induced by this antibiotic. In particular, data about the induction of stable CAs (translocations, inversions) by STZ will be useful to determine the long-term clastogenic effect of this compound.

At the molecular level, data obtained using the DNA microarray technology show that STZ induces changes (up- or down-regulation) in the expression of genes involved in different mammalian cellular processes [68,69]. However, the scarcity of reports on this issue indicates that further studies are needed to fully understand the regulation of gene expression by this antibiotic in mammalian cells.

Moreover, the scarcity of data available about the mutagenic and carcinogenic properties of STZ indicates that further intensive work needs to be done on these areas of research. In effect, little is known about the mutational spectra of STZ and the nature of the mutations induced by this antibiotic. Indeed, data on the carcinogenic effects of STZ on humans are still unavailable.

Finally, although the role of chemotherapy for neuroendocrine tumors remains controversial and no standard regimen has been proved to be effective [13-19], there have been several reports during recent years on the chemotherapeutic use of STZ which show that this antibiotic, in combination with several antineoplastic drugs and/or radiation can be used for the treatment of pancreatic neuroendocrine carcinomas. This issue opens a completely new horizon in the use of STZ as antineoplastic agent. However, the lack of efficacy of a STZ-based chemotherapeutic regimen in some patients with endocrine tumors shows that, in some cases, an alternative therapy must be applied.

## ACKNOWLEDGMENTS

Publications from the author, quoted in the present chapter, were supported by grants from the Consejo Nacional de Investigaciones Científicas y Técnicas (CONICET), the Comisión de Investigaciones Científicas de la Provincia de Buenos Aires (CICPBA), and Fundación Antorchas of Argentina.

## REFERENCES

[1] Lewis, C. & Barbiers, A. R. (1959/1960). Streptozotocin, a new antibiotic. *In vitro and in vivo* evaluation. *Antibiot. Ann.*, *7*, 247-254.

[2] Herr, R. R., Jahnke, A. D. & Argoudelis, A. D. (1967). The structure of Streptozotocin. *J. Am. Chem. Soc.*, *89*, 4808-4809.

[3] Raketien, N., Raketien, M. L. & Nadkarmi, M. (1963). Studies on the diabetogenic action of Streptozotocin. *Cancer Chemother. Rep.*, *29*, 91-98.

[4] Pisarev, V. B., Singur, G. L., Spasov, A. A., Samokhina, M. P. & Bulanov, A. E. (2009). Mechanisms of toxic effect of streptozotocin on β-cells in the islets of Langerhans. *Bull. Exp. Biol. Med.*, *148*, 937-939.

[5] Szkudelski, T. (2001). The mechanism of alloxan and streptozotocin action in β-cells of the rat pancreas. *Physiol. Res.*, *50*, 537-546.

[6] Szkudelski, T. (2012). The mechanism of alloxan and streptozotocin action in β-cells of the rat pancreas. *Exp. Biol. Med.*, *237*, 481-490.

[7] Reddy, S., Chang, M. & Robinson, E. (2006). Young NOD mice *Ann. New York Acad. Sci.*, *1079*, 109-113.

[8] Koulmanda, M., Qipo, A., Chebrolu, S., O'Neil, J., Auchincloss, H. & Smith, R. N. (2003). The effect of low versus high dose of streptozotocin in cynomolgus monkeys (Macaca fascilularis). *Am. J. Transplant*, *3*, 267-272.

[9] Rood, P. P., Bottino, R., Balamurugan, A. N., Smetanka, C., Ezzelarab, M., Busch, J., Hara, H., Trucco, M. & Cooper, D. K. (2006). Induction of diabetes *Pancreas*, *33*, 287-292.

[10] Prestayko, A. W., Crooke, S. T., Baker, L. H., Carter, S. K. & Schein. P. S. (Eds.). (1981). Nitrosoureas: Current Status and New Developments. *Academic Press*, *London.*

[11] Colvin, M. & Chabner, B. A. (1990). Alkylating Agents, in: Chabner, B.A. and Collins, J.M. (Eds.). Cancer Chemotherapy Principles and Practice. *J.B. Lippincott, Philadelphia*, 276-313.

[12] McConnick, J. E. & McElhinney, R. S. (1990). Nitrosoureas from chemist to physician: classification and recent approaches to drug design. *Eur. J. Cancer*, *26*, 207-221.

[13] Delaunoit, T., Ducreux, M., Boige, V., Dromain, C., Sabourin, J. C., Duvillard, P., Schlumberger, M. et al. (2004). The doxorubicin-streptozotocin combination for the treatment *Eur. J. Cancer*, *40*, 515-520.

[14] Strosberg, J. R., Hoffe, S., Gardner, N., Choi, J. & Kvols, L. (2007). Effective treatment *Neuroendocrinology*, *85*, 216-220.

[15] Turner, N. C., Strauss, S. J., Sarker, D., Gillmore, R., Kirkwood, A., Hackshaw, A., Papadopoulou, A. et al. (2010). Chemotherapy with 5-fluorouracil, cisplatin and streptozocin for neuroendocrine tumours *Br. J. Cancer*, *102*, 1106-1112.

[16] Chan, J. A. & Kulke, M. H. (2007). Emerging therapies for the treatment *Expert. Opin. Emerg. Drugs*, *12*, 253-270.

[17] Saif, M. W. (2011). Pancreatic neoplasm in 2011: an update. *JOP*, *12*, 316-321.

[18] Fassnacht, M., Terzolo, M., Allolio, B., Baudin, E., Haak, H., Berruti, A., Welin, S. et al. (2012). Combination chemotherapy in advanced adrenocortical carcinoma. *N. Engl. J. Med.*, *366*, 2189-2197.

[19] Reidy-Lagunes, D. L. (2012). Systemic therapy for advanced pancreatic neuroendocrine tumors: an update. *J. Natl. Compr. Canc. Netw.*, *10*, 777-783.

[20] Dolan, M. E. (1997). Inhibition of DNA repair as a means of increasing the antitumor activity of DNA reactive agents. *Adv. Drug Del. Rev.*, *26*, 105-118.

[21] Pegg, A. E. (1990). Mammalian $O^6$-alkylguanine-DNA-alkyltransferase: regulation and importance in response to alkylating carcinogenic and therapeutic agents. *Cancer Res.*, *50*, 6119-6129.

[22] Capucci, M. S., Hoffmann, M. E. & Natarajan, A. T. (1995). Streptozotocin-induced genotoxic effects in Chinese hamster cells: the resistant phenotype of V79 cells. *Mutat. Res.*, *347*, 79-85.

[23] Yang, H. & Wright, J. R. Jr. (2002). Human beta cells are exceedingly resistant to streptozotocin in vivo. *Endocrinology*, *143*, 2491-2495.

[24] Fazio, E. N. & Pin, C. L. (2007). Mist1-null mice are resistant to streptozotocin-induced beta cell damage. *Biochem. Biophys. Res. Commun.*, *353*, 823-828.

[25] Arison, R. N. & Feudale, E. L. (1967). Induction of renal tumour by Streptozotocin in rats. *Nature*, *214*, 1254-1255.

[26] Rakieten, N., Gordon, B. S., Cooney, D. A., Davis, R. D. & Schein, P. S. (1968). Renal tumorigenic action of Streptozotocin in rats. *Cancer Chemother. Rep.*, *52*, 563-567.

[27] Rakieten, N., Gordon, B. S., Beaty, A., Cooney, D. A., Davis, R. D. & Schein, P. S. (1971). Pancreatic islet cell tumors produced by the combined action of Streptozotocin and nicotinamide. *Proc. Soc. Exp. Biol. Med.*, *137*, 280-283.

[28] Rakieten, N., Gordon, B. S., Beaty, A., Cooney, D. A. & Schein, P. S. (1976). Modification of renal tumorigenic effect of Streptozotocin by nicotinarnide: spontaneous reversibiJity of Streptozotocin diabetes. *Proc. Soc. Exp. Biol. Med.*, *151*, 356-361.

[29] Iwase, M., Nunoi, K., Sadoshima, S., Kikuchi, M. & Fujishima, M. (1989). Liver, kidney and is let cell tumors in spontaneously hypertensive and normotensive rats treated with Streptozotocin. *Tohoku J. Exp. Med.*, *159*, 83-90.

[30] Weisburger, J. H., Griswold, D. P., Prejean, J. D., Casey, A. E., Wood, H. B. & Weisburger, E. K. (1975). The carcinogenic properties of some of the principal drugs used in clinical cancer chemotherapy. *Recent Results Cancer Res.*, *52*, 1-17.

[31] Vinerean, H. V., Gazda, L. S., Hall, R. D. & Smith, B. H. (2011). Streptozotocin is responsible for the induction and progression of renal tumorigenesis in diabetic Wistar-Furth rats treated with insulin or transplanted with agarose encapsulated porcine islets. *Islets*, *3*, 196-203.

[32] Sibay, T. M. & Hayes, J. A. (1969). Potential carcinogenic effect of Streptozotocin. *Lancet*, *2*, 912.

[33] Berman, L. D., Hayes, J. A. & Sibay, T. M. (1973). Effect of Streptozotocin in the Chinese hamster (*Cricetulus griseus*). *J. Natl. Cancer Inst.*, *51*, 1287-1294.

[34] Robbiano, L., Mereto, E., Corbu, C. & Brambilla, G. (1996). DNA damage induced by seven *N*-nitroso compounds in primary cultures of human and rat kidney cells. *Mutat. Res.*, *368*, 41-47.

[35] International Agency for Research on Cancer (IARC). (1978). Monographs on the evaluation of the carcinogenic risk of chemicals to humans no. 17: some *N*-Nitroso Compounds, Streptozotocin, 337-345.

[36] International Agency for Research on Cancer (IARC). (1987). Monographs, (Suppl. 7), p. 72.

[37] Bolzán, A. D. & Bianchi, M. S. (2002). Genotoxicity of streptozotocin. *Mutat. Res.*, *512*, 121-134.

[38] Tjälve, H. (1983). Streptozotocin: distribution, metabolism and mechanisms of action. *Uppsala J. Med. Sci. Suppl.*, *39*, 145-157.

[39] Bennett, R. A. & Pegg, A. E. (1981). Alkylation of DNA in rat tissues following administration of Streptozotocin. *Cancer Res.*, *41*, 2786-2790.

[40] Randerath, K., Reddy, M. V. & Gupta, R. C. (1981). $^{32}$P-labeling test for DNA damage. *Proc. Natl. Acad. Sci. U.S.A.*, *78*, 6126-6129.

[41] Day, R. S., Babich, M. A., Yarosh, D. B. & Scudiero, D. A. (1987). The role of $O^6$-methylguanine in human cell killing, sister chromatid exchange induction and mutagenesis: a review. *J. Cell Sci.*, *6 (Suppl.)*, 333-353.

[42] Margison, G. P. & O'Connor, P. J. (1990). Biological consequences of reactions with DNA: role of specific lesions. In: Cooper, C.S. and Grover, P.L. (Eds.), *Handbook of Experimental Pharmacology 94/1, Springer, Berlin*, 547-571.

[43] Pegg, A. E., Dolan, M. E. & Moschel, R. C. Structure, function, and inhibition of $O^6$-alkylguanine-DNA alkyltransferase. *Prog. Nucleic Acid Res. Mol. Biol.*, *51*, 167-223.

[44] Capucci, M. S., Hoffmann, M. E., De Groot, A. & Natarajan, A. T. (1995). Streptozotocin-induced toxicity in CHO-9 and V79 cells. *Environ. Mol. Mutagen.*, *26*, 72-78.

[45] Pegg, A. E., Wiest, L., Foote, R. S., Mitra, S. & Perry, W. (1983). Purification and properties of $O^6$-methylguanine-DNA transmethylase from rat liver. *J. Biol. Chem.*, *258*, 2327-2333.

[46] Saffhill, R., Margison, G. P. & O'Connor, P. J. (1985). Mechanisms of carcinogenesis induced by alkylating agents. *Biochim. Biophys. Acta*, *823*, 111-145.

[47] Loeb, L. A. (1985). Apurinic sites as mutagenic intermediates. *Cell*, *40*, 483-484.

[48] Erickson, L. C., Bradley, M. O. & Kohn, K. W. (1978). Measurements of DNA damage in Chinese hamster cells treated with equitoxic and equimutagenic doses of nitrosoureas. *Cancer Res.*, *38*, 3379-3384.

[49] Brambilla, G., Carlo, P., Finollo, R. & Sciaba, L. (1987). Dose-response curves for liver DNA fragmentation induced in rats by 16 *N*-nitroso compounds as measured by viscometric and alkaline elution analyses. *Cancer Res.*, *47*, 3485-3491.

[50] Petzold, G. L. & Swenberg, J. A. (1978). Detection of DNA damage induced in vivo following exposure of rats to carcinogens. *Cancer Res.*, *38*, 1589-1594.

[51] Yamamoto, H., Uchigata, Y. & Okamoto, H. (1981). Streptozotocin and alloxan induced DNA strand breaks and poly(ADPribose)synthetase in pancreatic islets. *Nature*, *294*, 284-286.

[52] Okamoto, H., Yarnamoto, H. & Uchigata, Y. (1982). Protection by superoxide dismutase, catalase and poly(ADP-ribose)synthetase inhibitors against alloxan-and Streptozotocin-induced islet DNA strand breaks and against proinsulin synthesis inhibition. In: Alberti, K.G., Ogada, T., Alouch, J.A.A. and Mngola, E.N. (Eds.), *Proceedings of 11th Congress International Diabetes Federation, Excerpta Medica, Amsterdam*, p. 13.

[53] Uchigata, Y., Yamamoto, H., Kavamura, A. & Okamoto, H. (1982). Protection by superoxide dismutase, catalase, and poly(ADP-ribose)synthetase inhibitors against alloxan-and Streptozotocin-induced islet DNA strand breaks and against the inhibition of proinsulin synthesis. *J. Biol. Chem.*, *257*, 6084.

[54] LeDoux, S. P., Woodley, S. E., Patton, N. J. & Wilson, G. L. (1986). Mechanisms of nitrosourea-induced -cell damage. Alterations in DNA. *Diabetes*, *35*, 866-872.

[55] Schmezer, P., Eckert, C. & Liegibel, U. M. (1994). Tissue-specific induction of mutations by Streptozotocin in vivo. *Mutat. Res.*, *307*, 495-499.

[56] Imaeda, A., Kaneko, T., Aoki, T., Kondo, Y. & Nagase, H. (2002). DNA *Food Chem. Toxicol.*, *40*, 979-987.

[57] Błasiak, J., Sikora, A., Wozniak, K. & Drzewoski, J. (2004). Genotoxicity of streptozotocin in normal and cancer cells and its modulation by free radical scavengers. *Cell Biol. Toxicol.*, *20*, 83-96.

[58] Nesslany, F., Zennouche, N., Simar-Meintières, S., Talahari, I., Nkili-Mboui, E. N. & Marzin, D. (2007). In vivo Comet assay on isolated kidney cells to distinguish

genotoxic carcinogens from epigenetic carcinogens or cytotoxic compounds. *Mutat. Res.*, *630*, 28-41.

[59] Kushwaha, S., Vikram, A., Trivedi, P. P. & Jena, G. B. (2011). Alkaline, Endo III and FPG modified comet assay as biomarkers for the detection of oxidative DNA damage in rats with experimentally induced diabetes. *Mutat. Res.*, *726*, 242-250.

[60] Lima, P. H., Sinzato, Y. K., Gelaleti, R. B., Calderon, I. M., Rudge, M. V. & Damasceno, D. C. (2012). Genotoxicity evaluation in severe or mild diabetic pregnancy in laboratory animals. *Exp. Clin. Endocrinol. Diabetes*, *120*, 303-307.

[61] Mossman, B. T., Ireland, C. M., Filipak, M., LeDoux, S. & Wilson, G. L. (1986). Comparative interactions of Streptozotocin and chlorozotocin with DNA of an insulin-secreting cell line (RINr). *Diabetologia*, *29*, 186-191.

[62] Pettepher, C. C., LeDoux, S. P., Bohr, V. A. & Wilson, G. L. (1991). Repair of alkali-labile sites within the mitochondrial DNA of RINr 38 cells after exposure to the nitrosourea Streptozotocin. *J. Biol. Chem.*, *266*, 3113-3117.

[63] Fram, R. J., Mack, S. L., George, M. & Marinus, M. G. (1989). DNA repair mechanisms affecting cytotoxicity by Streptozotocin in *E. coli*. *Mutat. Res.*, *218*, 125-133.

[64] Kraynak, A. R., Storer, R. D., Jensen, R. D., Kloss, M. W., Soper, K. A., Clair, J. H., DeLuca, J. G., Nichols, W. W. & Eydelloth, R. S. (1995). Extent and persistence of Streptozotocin-induced DNA damage and cell proliferation in rat kidney as determined by in vivo alkaline elution and BrdUrd labeling assays. *Toxicol. Appl. Pharmacol.*, *135*, 279-286.

[65] Tyson, C. K. & Mirsalis, J. C. (1985). Measurement of unscheduled DNA synthesis in rat kidney cells following in vivo treatment with genotoxic agents, *Environ. Mutagen.*, *7*, 889-899.

[66] Shepherd, J., Tsao, M. S. & Duguid, W. P. (1990). Genotoxicity of pancreatic chemical carcinogens to propagable cultured normal pancreatic epithelial cells. *Exp. Mol. Pathol.*, *53*, 203-210.

[67] Eizirik, D. L., Bjorklund, A. & Cagliero, E. (1993). Genotoxic agents increase expression of growth arrest and DNA damage-inducible genes *gadd* 153 and *gadd* 45 in rat pancreatic islets. *Diabetes*, *42*, 738-745.

[68] Kume, E., Aruga, C., Ishizuka, Y., Takahashi, K., Miwa, S., Itoh, M., Fujimura, H., Toriumi, W., Kitamura, K. & Doi, K. (2005). Gene expression profiling in streptozotocin treated mouse liver *Exp. Toxicol. Pathol.*, *56*, 235-244.

[69] Kume, E., Aruga, C., Takahashi, K., Miwa, S., Dekura, E., Itoh, M., Ishizuka, Y., Fujimura, H., Toriumi, W. & Doi, K. (2005). Morphological and gene expression *Exp. Toxicol. Pathol.* *56*, 245-253.

[70] Morgan, N. G., Cable, H. C., Newcombe, N. R. & Williams, G. T. (1994). Treatment of cultured pancreatic cells with Streptozotocin induces cell death by apoptosis. *Biosci. Rep.*, *14*, 243-250.

[71] Saini, K. S., Thompson, C., Winterford, C. M., Walker, N. I. & Cameron, D. P. (1996). Streptozotocin at low doses induces apoptosis and at high doses causes necrosis in a murine pancreatic -cell line, INS-1. *Biochem. Mol. Biol. Int.*, *39*, 1229-1236.

[72] Harel, A., Bloch, O., Vardi, P. & Bloch, K. (2002). Sensitivity of HaCat keratinocytes to diabetogenic toxins. *Biochem. Pharmacol.*, *63*, 171-178.

[73] Carpenter, L., Cordery, D. & Biden, T. J. (2002). Inhibition of protein kinase C delta protects rat INS-1 cells against interleukin-1beta and streptozotocin-induced apoptosis. *Diabetes*, *51*, 317-324.

[74] Hartley, J. A. & Gibson, N. W. (1986). DNA damage and cytotoxicity of 2-chloroethyl (methyllsulfonyl) methanesulfonate (NSC 338947) produced in human colon carcinoma cells with methylating agent pretreatment. *Cancer Res.*, *46*, 3871-3875.

[75] Gibson, N. W., Hartley, J. A., Barnes, D. & Erickson, L. C. (1986). Combined effects of strteptozotocin and mitozolomide against four human cell lines of the $Mer^+$ phenotype. *Cancer Res.*, *46*, 4995-4998.

[76] Murata, M., Takahashi, A., Saito, I. & Kawanishi, S. (1999). Site-specific DNA methylation and apoptosis: induction by diabetogenic Streptozotocin. *Biochem. Pharmacol.*, *57*, 881-887.

[77] Nukatsuka, M., Sakurai, H., Yoshimura, Y., Nishida, M. & Kawada, J. (1988). Enhancement by Streptozotocin of $O_2^-$ radical generation by the xanthine oxidase system of pancreatic cells. *FEBS Lett.*, *239*, 295-298.

[78] Kawada, J. (1992). New hypotheses for the mechanisms of Streptozotocin and alloxan inducing diabetes mellitus. *Yakugaku Zasshi*, *112*, 773-791.

[79] Takasu, N., Komiya, T., Asawa, T., Nagasawa, Y. & Yamada, T. (1991). Streptozotocin-and alloxan-induced $H_2O_2$ generation and DNA fragmentation in pancreatic islets. $H_2O_2$ as mediator for DNA fragmentation. *Diabetes*, *40*, 1141-1145.

[80] Ohkuwa, T., Sato, Y. & Naoi, M. (1995). Hydroxyl radical formation in diabetic rats induced by Streptozotocin. *Life Sci.*, *56*, 1789-1798.

[81] Bedoya, F. J., Solano, F. & Lucas, M. (1996). *N*-monomethyl-arginine and nicotinamide prevent Streptozotocin-induced double strand DNA break formation in pancreatic rat islets. *Experientia*, *52*, 344-347.

[82] Kroncke, K. D., Fehsel, K., Sommer, A., Rodriguez, M. L. & Kolb-Bachofen, V. (1995). Nitric oxide generation during cellular metabolization of the diabetogenic *N*-methyl-*N*-nitroso-urea streptozotozin contributes to islet cell DNA damage. *Biol. Chem. Hoppe Seyler.*, *376*, 179-185.

[83] Chen, H., Carlson, E. C., Pellet, L., Moritz, J. T. & Epstein, P. N. (2001). Overexpression of metallothionein in pancreatic cell reduces Streptozotocin-induced DNA damage and diabetes. *Diabetes*, *50*, 2040-2046.

[84] Gandy, S. E., Buse, M. G. & Crouch, R. K. (1982). Protective role of superoxide dismutase against diabetogenic drugs. *Clin. Res.*, *30*, 392a.

[85] Robbins, M. J., Sharp, R. A., Slonim, A. E. & Burr, I. M. (1980). Protection against Streptozotocin-induced diabetes by superoxide dismutase. *Diabetologia*, *18*, 55.

[86] Gandy, S. E., Buse, M. G., Sorenson, J. R. J. & Crouch, R. K. (1983). Attenuation of Streptozotocin diabetes with superoxide dismutase-1ike copper (nX3,5-diisopropylsalicylate) in the rat. *Diabetologia*, *24*, 437.

[87] Sandler, S. & Andersson, A. (1982). The partial protection effect of the hydroxyl radical scavenger dimethylurea on Streptozotocin-induced diabetes *in vivo and in vitro*. *Diabetologia*, *23*, 374.

[88] Slonim, A. E., Surber, M. E., Page, D. E., Sharp, R. A. & Burr, I. M. (1983). Modification of chernically induced diabetes in rats by Vitamin E: supplementation minimizes and depletion enhances development of diabetes. *J. Clin. Invest.*, *71*, 1282.

[89] Imaeda, A., Kaneko, T., Aoki, T., Kondo, Y., Nakamura, N., Nagase, H. & Yoshikawa, T. (2002). Antioxidative effects of fluvastatin and its metabolites *Food Chem. Toxicol. 40*, 1415-1422.

[90] Wayhs, C. A., Manfredini, V., Sitta, A., Deon, M., Ribas, G. S., Vanzin, C. S., Biancini, G. B., Nin, M. S., Barros, H. M. & Vargas, C. R. (2010). Effects of insulin and clonazepam on DNA damage in diabetic rats submitted to the forced swimming test. *Mutat. Res., 703*, 187-190.

[91] Bhuyan, B. K. (1969). Action of Streptozotocin, an antileukemic antibiotic, on L1210 cells. In: P. Farnes (Ed.), *In Vitro Vol. 4, Baltimore, The Williams and Wilkins Co.*, p. 154.

[92] Kelly, F. & Legator, M. (1971). The effects of *N*-methyl-*N*-nitro*N*-nitrosoguanidine and Streptozotocin on mammalian cell cultures. *Mutat. Res., 12*, 183-190.

[93] Capucci, M. S., Hoffmann, M. E., Zdzienicka, M. Z. & Natarajan, A. T. (1995). Streptozotocin-induced chromosomal aberrations, SCEs and mutations in CHO-9 parental cells and in EM-C11 mutant cell line. *Mutat. Res., 326*, 227-234.

[94] Bolzán, A. D., Bianchi, N. O. & Bianchi, M. S. (1998). Effects of antioxidants on Streptozotocin-induced clastogenesis in mammalian and insect cells. *Mutat. Res., 418*, 35-42.

[95] Bolzán, A. D., González, M. C. & Bianchi, M. S. (2000). The effect of 1,10-phenanthroline on the chromosome damage and sister-chromatid exchanges induced by Streptozotocin in mammalian and insect cells. *Mutat. Res., 447*, 221-226.

[96] Bolzán, A. D. & Bianchi, M. S. (2002). Chromosomal response of human lymphocytes to Streptozotocin. *Mutat. Res., 503*, 63-68.

[97] Bhuyan, B. K. (1970). The action of Streptozotocin on mammalian cells. *Cancer Res., 30*, 2017-2023.

[98] Kaina, B. (1987). Correction of alkylation hypersensitivity of CHO-W27-1 by transfection with human DNA. *Carcinogenesis, 11*, 1209-1212.

[99] Kaina, B., Ziouta, A., Ochs, K. & Coquerelle, T. (1997). Chromosomal instability, cell death and apoptosis induced by $O^6$-methylguanine in Mex−, Mex+ and methylation-tolerant mismatch repair comprornised cells: facts and models. *Mutat. Res., 381*, 227-241.

[100] Kaina, B., Fritz, G. & Coquerelle, T. (1993). Contribution of $O^6$-alkylguanine and *N*-alkylpurines to the formation of sister chromatid exchanges, chromosomal aberrations, and gene mutations: new insights gained from studies of genetically engineered mammalian cell lines. *Environ. Mol. Mutagen., 22*, 283-292.

[101] Bolzán, A. D. & Bianchi, M. S. (2003). Clastogenic effects of Streptozotocin on human colon cancer cell lines. *J. Environ. Pathol. Toxicol. Oncol., 22*, 281-286.

[102] Liegibel, U., Tinwell, H., Callander, R. D., Schmezer, P. & Ashby, J. (1992). Clastogenicity to the mouse bone marrow of the mouse germ cell genotoxin Streptozotocin. *Mutagenesis, 7*, 471-474.

[103] Chinnasamy, N., Fairbairn, L. J., Laher, J., Willington, M. A. & Rafferty, J. A. (1998). Modulation of $O^6$-alkylating agent induced clastogenicity by enhanced DNA repair capacity of bone marrow cells. *Mutat. Res., 416*, 1-10.

[104] Tokuda, K. & Bodell, W. J. (1998) Cytotoxicity and induction of sister chromatid exchanges in human and rodent brain tumor cells treated with alkylating chemotherapeutic agents. *Cancer Res., 48*, 3100-3105.

[105] Vikram, A., Tripathi, D. N., Ramarao, P. & Jena, G. B. (2007). Evaluation of streptozotocin genotoxicity in rats from different ages using the micronucleus assay. *Regul. Toxicol. Pharmacol.*, *49*, 238-244.

[106] Bolzán, A. D. & Bianchi, M. S. (2005). Analysis of streptozotocin-induced incomplete chromosome elements and excess acentric fragments in Chinese hamster cells using a telomeric PNA probe. *Mutat. Res.*, *570*, 237-244.

[107] Quiroga, I. Y., Paviolo, N. S. & Bolzán, A. D. (2013). Effect of the methylating agent streptozotocin on interstitial telomeric sequences. *Environ. Mol. Mutagen.*, *54*, 147-152.

[108] Day III, R. S., Ziolkowski, C. H. J., Scudiero, D. A., Meyer, S. A., Libiniecki, A. S., Girardi, A. J., Galloway, S. M. & Bynum, G. D. (1980). Defective repair of alkylated DNA by human tumor and SV-40 transformed human cell strains. *Nature*, *288*, 724-727.

[109] Goldmaker, V. S., Cuzich, R. A. & Thilly, W. G. (1986). Isolation and partial characterization of human cell mutants differing in sensitivity to killing and mutation of methylnitrosourea and *N*-methyl-*N*′-nitro-*N*-nitrosoguanidine. *J. Biol. Chem.*, *261*, 12462-12471.

[110] Goth-Goldstein, R. & Hughes, M. (1987). Characterization of a CHO variant in respect to alkylating agent-induced biological effects and DNA repair. *Mutat. Res.*, *184*, 139-146.

[111] Galloway, S. M., Greenwood, S. K., Hill, R. B., Bradt, C. I. & Bean, C. L. (1995). A role for mismatch repair in production of chromosome aberrations by methylating agents in human cells. *Mutat. Res.*, *346*, 231-245.

[112] Zlotogorski, C. & Erickson, L. C. (1983). Pretreatrnent of normal human fibroblasts and human colon carcinoma cells with MNNG allows chloroethylnitrosourea to produce DNA interstrand crosslinks not observed in cells treated with chloroethylnitrosourea alone. *Carcinogenesis*, *4*, 759-763.

[113] Zeller, W. J., Berger, M. R., Henne, T. & Weber, E. (1986). More than additive toxicity of the combination of 1-methyl-1nitrosourea plus 1,3-bis(2-chloroethyl)-I-nitrosourea in the rat. *Cancer Res.*, *46*, 1714-1716.

[114] Futscher, B. W., Micetich, K. C., Barnes, D. M., Fisher, R. I. & Erickson, L. C. (1989). Inhibition of a specific DNA repair system and nitrosourea cytotoxicity in resistant human cancer cells. *Cancer Commun.*, *1*, 65-73.

[115] Pieper, R. O., Futscher, B. W., Dong, Q. & Erickson, L. C. (1991). Effects of Streptozotocin/bis-chloroethylnitrosourea combination therapy on $O^6$-methylguanine DNA methyltransferase activity and mRNA levels in HT-29 cells in vitro. *Cancer Res.*, *51*, 1581-1585.

[116] Tokuda, K. (1992). Effect of pretreatment with *N*-methyl-*N*nitrosourea or Streptozotocin on the cytotoxicity and the induction of sister chromatid exchanges in human and rodent brain tumor cells treated with chloroethylnitrosourea. *Hokkaido Igaku Zasshi*, *67*, 462-474.

[117] Ishida, R. and Takahashi, T. (1987). *N*-methyl-*N*′-nitrosoguanidineresistant Hela S3 cells still have little $O^6$-methylguanine-DNA-methyltransferase activity and are hypermutable by alkylating agents. *Carcinogenesis (London)*, *8*, 1109-1113.

[118] Samson, L. & Linn, S. (1987). Alkylation repair and the induction of cell death and sister chromatid exchange in human cells. *Carcinogenesis (London)*, *8*, 227-230.

[119] Aquilina, G., Zijno, A., Moscufo, N., Dogliotti, N. E. & Bignami, M. (1989). Tolerance to methylniytosourea-induced DNA damage is associated with 6-thioguanine res´ıstanse in CHO cells. *Carcinogenesis*, *10*, 1219-1223.

[120] Godfrey, D. B., Bouffler, S. D., Musk, S. R. R., Raman, M. J. & Johnson, R. T. (1992). Mammalian cells share a common pathway for the relief of DNA replication arrest by $O^6$-alkylguanine, incorporated 6-thioguanine and UV photoproducts. *Mutat. Res.*, *274*, 225-235.

[121] Ishida, R. & Utsumi, K. R. (1990). Differences in induction of sister chromatid exchange in MNNG-resistant HeLa S3-Mer-cell lines. *Carcinogenesis*, *11*, 1209-1212.

[122] Mello-Filho, A. & Meneghini, R. (1985). Protection of mammalian cells by *o*-phenanthroline from lethal and DNA-damaging effects produced by active oxygen species. *Biochim. Biophys. Acta*, *847*, 82-89.

[123] Eizirik, D. L., de Lucio, M. A., Boschero, A. C. & Hoffmann, M. E. (1986). 1,10 Phenanthroline, a metal chelator, protects against alloxan-but not Streptozotocin-induced diabetes. *J. Free Radic. Biol. Med.*, *2*, 189-192.

[124] Kaina, B. (1998). Critical steps in alkylation-induced aberration formation. *Mutat. Res.*, *404*, 119-124.

[125] Kolbye, S. M. & Legator, M. S. (1968). Mutagenic activity of Streptozotocin. *Mutat. Res.*, *6*, 387-389.

[126] Ficsor, G. & Muthiani, E. (1971). A microbial assay for detecting chemical mutagens in tissue homogenates. *Mutat. Res.*, *12*, 335-337.

[127] McCann, J., Choi, E., Yamasaki, E. & Ames, B. N. (1975). Detection of carcinogens as mutagens in the *Salmonella*/microsome test: assay of 300 chemicals. *Proc. Natl. Acad. Sci. U.S.A.*, *72*, 5135-5139.

[128] Zimmer, D. M. & Bhuyan, B. K. (1976). Mutagenicity of Streptozotocin and several other nitrosourea compounds in *Salmonella typhimurium*. *Mutat. Res.*, *40*, 281-288.

[129] Ficsor, G., Bordas, S. & Stewart, S. J. (1978). Mutagenicity testing of benomyl, methyl-2-benzimidazole carbamate, Streptozotocin and *N*-methyl-*N'*-nitro-*N*-nitrosoguanidine in *Salmonella typhimurium* in vitro and in rodent host-mediated assays. *Mutat. Res.*, *51*, 151-164.

[130] Franza Jr., B. R., Oeschger, N. S., Oeschger, M. P. & Schein, P. S. (1980). Mutagenic activity of nitrosourea antitumor agents. *J. Natl. Cancer Inst.*, *65*, 149-154.

[131] Fram, R. J., Sullivan, J. & Marinus, M. G. (1986). Mutagenesis and repair of DNA damage caused by nitrogen mustard, *N,N'*bis(2-chloroethyl)-*N*-nitrosourea (BCNU), Streptozotocin and mitomycin C in *E. coli*. *Mutat. Res.*, *66*, 299-342.

[132] Marczewska, J. & Koziorowska, J. (1997). Comparison of the induction of SOS repair in *Escherichia coli* PQ37 and PQ243 by antineoplastic agents. *Acta Pol. Pharm.*, *54*, 35-41.

[133] Lengeler, J. (1980). Characterisation of mutants of *Escherichia coli* K12, selected by resistance to Streptozotocin. *Mol. Gen. Genet.*, *179*, 49-54.

[134] Gabridge, M. G., Denunzio, A. & Legator, M. S. (1969). Microbial mutagenicity of Streptozotocin in animal-mediated assays. *Nature*, *221*, 68-70.

[135] Bhuyan, B. K., Peterson, A. R. & Heidelberger, C. (1976). Cytotoxicity, mutations and DNA damage produced in Chinese hamster cells treated with Streptozotocin, its analogs, and *N*-methyl-*N'*-nitro-*N*-nitrosoguanidine. *Chem. Biol. Interact.*, *13*, 173-179.

[136] Browning, L. S. (1973). Mutagenicity of various chemicals and their metabolites in *Drosophila*. *Genetics*, *74*, 33 [abstract].

[137] Rodríguez-Arnaiz, R. & Aranda, J. H. (1994). Metabolic activation of four drugs in the eye mosaic assay measuring principally mitotic recombination in *Drosophila melanogaster*: differences in strain susceptibility and route of exposure. *Mutat. Res.*, *305*, 157-163.

[138] Hernando, J., Álvarez, L., Ferreiro, J. A., Sancho, I., Comendador, M. A. & Sierra, L. M. (2004). Female germ cell mutagenicity of model chemicals in Drosophila melanogaster: mechanistic information and analysis of repair systems. *Mutat. Res.*, *545*, 59-72.

[139] Araki, A., Sasaki, T. & Matsushima, T. (2008). Comparison of sensitivity of Escherichia coli WP2 tester strains with and without tolC outer membrane transport protein mutation in detecting chemical mutagens. *J. UOEH*, *30*, 133-145.

In: Streptozotocin: Uses, Mechanism of Action and Side Effects ISBN: 978-1-63117-255-7
Editor: Elizabeth L. Gauthier 

*Chapter 7*

# TOXIC EFFECT OF STREPTOZOTOCIN (STZ) ON THE HEPATOBILIARY FUNCTION: OXIDATIVE STRESS AND INFLAMMATION MAY CONTRIBUTE TO THE HEPATIC COMPLICATIONS DURING STZ-INDUCED INSULIN-DEPENDENT DIABETES

***C. E. Carnovale[1,2,*], D. E. Francés[1], P. I. Ingaramo[1] and M. T. Ronco[1]***

[1]Instituto de Fisiología Experimental (CONICET), Facultad de Ciencias Bioquímicas y Farmacéuticas (Universidad Nacional de Rosario), Rosario, Argentina
[2]Facultad de Ciencias de la Salud-Universidad Autónoma de Chile, Chile

## ABSTRACT

Streptozotocin (STZ: 2-deoxy-2-(3-(methyl-3-nitrosoureido)-D-glucopyranose) is synthesized by *Streptomycetes achromogenes* and is used to induce both insulin-dependent and non-insulin-dependent diabetes mellitus (IDDM and NIDDM, respectively).

The single intravenous dose most frequently used in adult rats to induce IDDM is between 40 and 60 mg/kg b.w., but higher doses are also used. STZ is also efficacious after intraperitoneal administration of a similar or higher dose.

Streptozotocin action on B cells is accompanied by characteristic alterations in the blood levels of insulin and glucose. Two hours after injection, hyperglycemia is observed together with a concomitant drop in blood insulin. About six hours later, hypoglycemia occurs with high levels of blood insulin. Finally, hyperglycemia develops and blood insulin levels decrease. These changes in the blood levels of glucose and insulin reflect abnormalities of B cell function. STZ impairs glucose oxidation and decreases insulin biosynthesis and secretion.

The liver plays an important role in the metabolism and excretion of STZ. At first, we analyzed the direct effect of STZ on the hepatobiliary function. The effect of

* E-mail: ccarnova@fbioyf.unr.edu.ar.

streptozotocin on hepatobiliary function was studied in rats on the 1$^{st}$, 7$^{th}$ and 15$^{th}$ days after treatment. Serum glucose significantly increased on the 1st day, and remained high onwards. Bile flow and the bile acids output were significantly decreased on the 1$^{st}$ day of treatment. Also, the biliary excretion of sulfobromophthalein (BSP, a substance used for evaluating the function of the liver) was significantly decreased on the first day of treatment. All parameters tested, except for serum glucose, tended to normalize at 7$^{th}$ day after treatment. The results suggested a transient toxic effect of STZ on the hepatocyte. It is known that bile flow (BF) is determined by two fractions: the bile acid dependent flow (BADF) and the bile acid independent flow (BAIF). We analyzed both fractions and demonstrated that STZ itself, and not its diabetogenic effect, produced a diminution in BF at the expense of both BAIF and BADF.

In a second stage, we used STZ to induce insulin-dependent diabetes in rats. It is known that the liver is a central regulator of carbohydrate homeostasis and it releases glucose according to metabolic demand. Besides, in the last years, liver injury has been recognized as a major complication of diabetes mellitus (DM).

We analyzed the contribution of oxidative stress and Tumor Necrosis Factor alpha (TNF-α) intracellular pathway in the development of apoptosis in the liver of streptozotocin- induced diabetic animals. In this review, we describe the role of upstream mediators of the interaction between TNFα and its receptor, TNFR1, by assessing the ability of the *in vivo* treatment with etanercept (TNF-α blocking antibody) to protect against TNF-α-induced apoptosis. Also, we studied the role of iNOS-induction in the TNF-α pathways of liver apoptosis in IDDM, by treatment of diabetic rats with aminoguanidine (selective iNOS inhibitor), which blocked the induction of apoptosis. Interestingly, iNOS inhibition significantly reduced TNF-α levels, thus evidencing an interaction between TNF-α and iNOS activity. On the other hand, we found that the administration of antioxidants/hydroxyl radical scavengers (Tempol and Desferal) prevented oxidative stress by reducing the effects of hydroxyl radical production and both LPO levels and apoptosis. Taken together, our studies support the notion that, at least in part, the hydroxyl radical acts as a reactive intermediate, which leads to liver apoptosis in a model of STZ-mediated hyperglycemia.

The present review bears two major insights:

First, it provides evidence for a transient toxic effect of STZ on the hepatobiliary function. This toxic effect becomes relevant for the study, at short time, of hepatic metabolism in the experimental diabetes induced by STZ.

Second, it provides further knowledge about the mechanisms which may contribute to the disease process in the liver during the course of an inflammatory process as is IDDM. Regulation of hepatic oxidative stress and TNF-α levels in the diabetic state could be of therapeutic relevance for the improvement or delay of the hepatic complications linked to chronic hyperglycemia.

**Keywords:** Streptozotocin, Bile Flow, Diabetes mellitus, Liver, Apoptosis, Inflammation, TNF-α, iNOS, NO, Oxidative stress, Hydroxyl radical

## INTRODUCTION

The induction of experimental diabetes in the rat using chemicals which selectively destroy pancreatic B cells is very convenient and simple to use. One of the most usual substances to induce diabetes in the rat is streptozotocin [1]. The understanding of the changes occurring in B cells of the pancreas as well as in the whole organism after streptozotocin treatment is essential for the use of this compound as a diabetogenic agent. The metabolic disturbances in streptozotocin-treated rats have been described by different authors [2-4]. This review focuses on two different aspects: First, it provides evidence for a transient toxic effect of STZ on the hepatobiliary function. This toxic effect becomes relevant for the study, at short time, of hepatic metabolism in the experimental diabetes induced by STZ. Second, it provides further knowledge about the mechanisms which may contribute to the disease process in the liver during the course of an inflammatory process as is IDDM when toxic effects of insulin have dissapeared.

Regulation of hepatic TNF-α levels and oxidative stress in the diabetic state could be of therapeutic relevance for the improvement or delay the hepatic complications linked to chronic hyperglycemia.

## 1. Mechanism of Streptozotocin Action on the Pancreatic B Cells

Streptozotocin (STZ, 2 – deoxy – 2 - (3 - (methyl - 3 -nitrosoureido) -D-glucopyranose) is synthesized by *Streptomycetes achromogenes* and is used to induce both insulin-dependent and non-insulin-dependent diabetes mellitus (IDDM and NIDDM, respectively).

The range of the STZ dose commonly used is broad. The single intravenous dose most frequently used in adult rats to induce IDDM is between 40 and 60 mg/kg b.w. [5], but higher doses are also used.

STZ is also efficacious after intraperitoneal administration of a similar or higher dose, but a single dose below 40 mg/kg b.w. may be ineffective [6]. For instance, when we injected 50 mg/kg b.w. STZ intravenously to Wistar rats, blood glucose (determined 2 weeks after treatment) can reach about 30 mM [7]. *A posteriori*, we also used 60 mg/kg b.w. STZ injected intraperitonealy to Wistar rats, and blood glucose (determined 2 weeks after treatment) reached about 26 mM [8].

NIDDM can easily be induced in rats by intravenous or intraperitoneal treatment with 100 mg/kg b.w. STZ on the day of birth. This method of NIDDM induction was described for the first time by Portha et al. (1974) [9]. At 8-10 weeks of age and thereafter, rats neonatally treated with STZ manifest mild basal hyperglycemia, an impaired response to the glucose tolerance test [10] and a loss of B cell sensitivity to glucose [11].

STZ is taken up by pancreatic B cells via glucose transporter GLUT2. Intracellular action of STZ results in changes of DNA in pancreatic B cells comprising its fragmentation [12]. Some experiments have proved that the main reason for the STZ-induced B cell death is alkylation of DNA, which contributes to its fragmentation [13]. On the other hand, STZ was found to generate reactive oxygen species (ROS), and when it is metabolized inside the cells, it liberates NO. The synergistic action of both NO and ROS may also contribute to DNA fragmentation [4].

STZ-induced DNA damage activates poly ADP- ribosylation [14] which leads to depletion of cellular NAD+, further reduction of the ATP content [15] and subsequent inhibition of insulin synthesis and secretion [16]. The concept of unfavorable consequences of augmented poly ADP-ribosylation as a result of STZ action was confirmed by experiments revealing that the inhibition of this process prevents the toxicity of this diabetogenic agent

[17]. Thus, it can be stated that the activation of poly ADP-ribosylation is of greater importance for the diabetogenicity of STZ than generation of free radicals and DNA damage *per se*.

# 2. Toxic Effect of STZ in the Liver Function

## 2.1. Liver Metabolism and Excretion of STZ: Studies of the Global Function of Liver

In studies performed with radiolabelled streptozotocin it was demonstrated that STZ is subject to partial metabolic transformation in the liver. Biliary and intestinal excretion of streptozotocin and its metabolites was also observed [18, 19].

Based on this previous knowledge, the aim of our studies was to determine if a diabetogenic dose of STZ, which induces IDDM in adult rats, also produce changes in the liver function.

We performed the studies in male Wistar rats, injected intravenously with a diabetogenic dose of STZ of 50 mg/kg b.w. (dissolved in 0.05 M citrate buffer). The control rats were injected with buffer alone. First, we carried out the studies 24 h, 7 days and 15 days after STZ injection (or citrate buffer in controls). On the day of the experiment, animals were anesthetized with sodium pentobarbital (50 mg/kg body weight, i.p.), the bile duct and femoral vein were cannulated, and the bile was collected. On the 1$^{st}$ day of STZ treatment serum glucose levels increased significantly. Hiperglycemia in 7-day and 15-day diabetic rats was about the same as on 1$^{st}$-day animals, about 20 mM. The serum sorbitol dehydrogenase activity, a sensitive indicator of liver damage [20], was markedly increased on the 1$^{st}$ day of the injection of STZ, and a clear tendency to return to the values obtained in the controls was observed on the 7$^{th}$ and 15$^{th}$ days post-injection.

On the other hand, the bile flow (BF) and the bile acid (BA) output were decreased significantly on the 1$^{st}$ day of STZ treatment. While the bile acid output showed a clear tendency to return to control values at the 7$^{th}$ day, bile flow decrease continued at this time, althought it was less pronounced. The results suggest that STZ administration to rats induced a transient impairment of the processes involved in bile formation. Since BA are considered to be one of the main solutes involved in the generation of BF [21, 22] we can asume that BA-dependent flow was impaired in STZ-treated rats. However, despite the fact that BA output was normalized on the 7$^{th}$ day of treatment, BF depression still continued, although it was less pronunced.

Thus, we can not discard the possibility that BA-independent flow, which is determined by the secretion into bile of both glutathione and bicarbonate anion [23, 24], was also altered by STZ administration.

To evaluate the global function of the liver, we performed the disodium sulfobromophthalein excretion test (BSP). BSP is a dye that is transported into hepatocytes by organic anion transporting polypeptides (OATPs) in sinusoidal membrane with high affinity, and after conjugation with glutathione, it is excreted into bile by the canalicular multidrug resistance associated protein 2 (Mrp2) [25-27]. BSP was given as a single femoral vein injection (60 mg/kg b.wt.) and bile samples were collected every 15 min for a 90-min period.

BSP biliary excretion was significantly delayed on the 1st day of STZ treatment but a pattern similar to that of controls was observed on days 7 and 15 post-injection. The proportion of conjugated BSP did not show differences between controls and treated rats. The results suggest that STZ administration to rats induced a transient impairment of the processes involved in bile formation [7].

## 2.2. Studies of the Bile Acid-Dependent and –Independent Fractions of Bile Flow

Later, we analysed the effect of STZ (on the 1st day of treatment) on the Bile Acid (BA)-dependent bile flow (BADF) and the BA-independent bile flow (BAIF). For this purpose, immediatly after cannulation of the bile duct, bile samples were collected for 60 min (basal period). An intravenous infusión of sodium taurocholate was started at the rate of 300 nmoles/min/100 g body w.t. BAIF was estimated by an extrapolation to zero time of the regression line between BF and BA secretion rate [28]. STZ produced a decrease in BF at the expense of both BAIF (-37%) and BADF (-39%) [29].

Bicarbonate anion ($HCO3^-$) is one of the determinants of BA-independent bile flow (BAIF) [24, 30]. Overall, $HCO3^-$ transport involves the sequential participation of three different transporters, namely $Na^+$, $K^+$- adenosine triphosphatase ($Na^+$, $K^+$- ATPase), NHE ($Na^+/H^+$ exchanger), localized at the basolateral domain, and AE2/Ae2 (anion exchanger 2; SLC4A2/slc4a2), localized at the apical domain. $Na^+$, $K^+$- ATPase activity maintains plasma-to-cytosol $Na^+$ gradients for basolateral efflux of $H^+$ via NHE. The extruded $H^+$ neutralizes $HCO3^-$ in plasma, enabling its passive diffusion as CO2. After conversion of CO2 back into $HCO3^-$ by intracellular carbonic anhydrase, the anion is counter-transported with $Cl^-$ at the canalicular domain by AE2/Ae2 [31].

In this connection, we have analysed the main factors involved in the impairment of formation of the BA-independent bile flow (BAIF) in streptozotocin (STZ)-treated rats. Twenty-four hours after STZ injection (50 mg/kg body wt, i.v.) BF, bile salt output and biliary excretion of the major inorganic electrolytes ($Na^+$, $Cl^-$, $HCO3^-$) were significantly decreased.

The relationship between bile flow and bile salt output obtained during the administration of sodium taurocholate at stepwise-increasing rates indicated that BAIF (y-intercept) was decreased by 37% in STZ-treated rats. The relationship between electrolyte output and bile salt output showed that the $Na^+$, $Cl^-$ and $HCO3^-$ fractions excreted independently of bile acid (y-intercept) decreased to 59%, 47% and 67% of the control values respectively, while the amount of electrolyte secreted per unit of bile acid secreted was unaffected in STZ-treated rats. The hepatic activity of $Na^+$, $K^+$- ATPase was decreased by 59% ($p<0.05$) in STZ-treated rats.

Nicotinamide is a compound whose intraperitoneal administration, in rats, at a single dose of 500mg/kg body wt prior to STZ injection, prevents the diabetogenic effect of this latter drug without concomitant loss of its antitumour activity [32]. We administered nicotinamide prior to STZ to prevent the hyperglycemia indicative of STZ-induced diabetes, and we observed no effect on the decrease in $Na^+$, $K^+$- ATPase activity. These results suggest that STZ itself, and not its diabetogenic effect, decreases the BAIF by a mechanism that involves impairment of the biliary electrolyte excretion, which could be the result of the inhibition of the hepatic $Na^+$, $K^+$- ATPase activity [33].

On the other hand, bile acids are the predominant organic solutes in bile and the main determinants of bile flow wich, specifically of the BADF. Conservation of the bile acid pool is facilitated by the efficient reabsorption of bile acids from the gastrointestinal tract. Absorption can take place by several mechanisms which mainly include passive nonionic diffusion and active transport [22, 34]. We studied the excretion of fecal bile acids in living rats injected with sodium [$^{14}$C] taurocholate (TC), and we observed an increase in BA fecal excretion in STZ-treated animals. This event could account for the decrease in the uptake of BA seen in our experiments *in vitro*. Everted distal ileum segments were prepared from non-fasted controls and STZ-treated rats at 24 h after the injection. The intestine was removed from pentobarbital-anaesthetized animals following a midline abdominal incision and transection of the intestine at the piloric and ileocecal junctions. The distal 11-cm segment was separated, rinsed in ice-cold 0.9% sodium chloride solution, everted with the use of a glass rod and positioned on the incubation chamber as reported previously [35]. The mucosal solution was cotinuosly bubbled with oxigen. The tissues underwent a 10-min preincubation period in the buffer before the addition of sodium taurocholate (0.1 μCi) to the mucosal medium (8 ml).

Total serosal fluid (1 ml) was collected at 2, 5, 10, 15 and 20 min, and replaced each time with fresh buffer within 20 s. Mucosal samples (0.2 ml) were collected at the same time periods. The active transport of TC was verified in control preparations from the serosal-to-mucosal ratio (S/M), which reached a value of 2 at 20 min of incubation in control rats. 24 h after STZ administration the concentrative transport was not observed, and the S/M ratio was lower than 1 at 20 min of incubation. The viability of the preparation used for *in vitro* experiments was evaluated by light microscopy and by the rate of tissue [$^{14}$C]-sucrose uptake from the mucosal fluid.

We observed that TC transfer to the serosal fluid was impaired after 24 h of STZ injection, and that the same occurred with the active transport in control preparations. The amount of TC accumulated in the intestinal tissue was also decreased. In addition, total ATPase activity was decreased, and intracellular electrolyte concentration was altered. Therefore, a slower saturation of binding sites could be responsible for the effects of STZ on TC tissue accumulation, and a decreased ATPase activity would account for the impairment of the TC concentrative transport system [36].

Stone J l et al. analysed the organic anion uptake in STZ-induced diabetes, and they concluded, in accordance with our results, that initial STZ toxicity may decrease bile flow until cellular repair occurs and cellular function returns to normal. However, by 7 days after STZ, organic anion uptake from the circulation and biliary excretion of bile acids are both increased over that of the normal animals, thus indicating that STZ toxicity is no longer an important factor affecting bile flow [37].

Figure 1 shows a schematic representation of the main STZ transient toxic effects demonstrated by our laboratory to bile flow formation at both bile acid-independent bile flow (BAIF) and bile salt -dependent bile flow (BADF).

In conclusion, the study of the hepatic function in the experimental diabetes induced by STZ should not be performed until the recovery of STZ-induced toxicity takes place (according to our studies, 15 days after administration STZ), to accurately analyze the alterations that occur in the diabetic state.

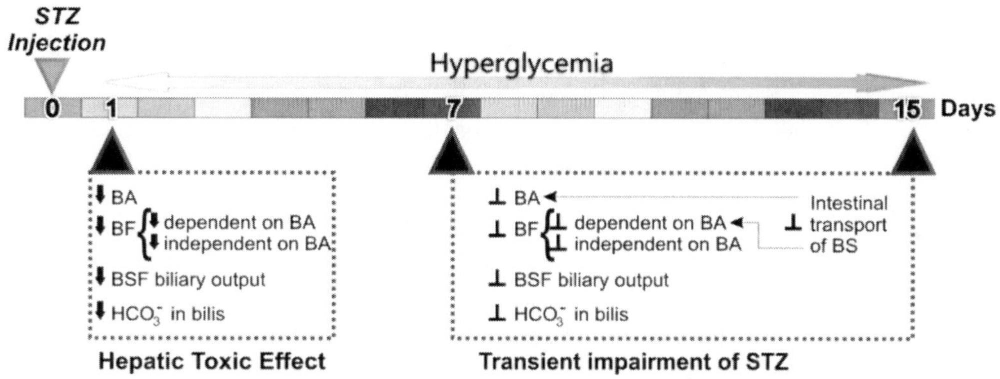


Figure 1. Schematic representation of the main STZ transient toxic effects demonstrated by our laboratory to bile flow formation at both bile acid-independent bile flow (BAIF) and bile acid - dependent bile flow (BADF). (⊥: return to the values obtained in the controls).

## 3. Oxidative Stress and Inflammation May Contribute to the Hepatic Complications during STZ-Induced Insulin-Dependent Diabetes

In our laboratory, STZ-induced (IDDM) was achieved by a single dose of STZ (60mg/kg b. w., i.p., in 50 mM citrate buffer, pH 4.5). Fifteen days after STZ injection, a time when the toxic effect of the drug on the liver has disappeared [7, 29], serum glucose levels were tested by means of the glucose oxidase method (Wiener Lab., Rosario, Argentina) in samples of diabetic and control animals. Successful induction of diabetes was defined as a blood glucose level higher than13.2 mM.

### 3.1. Oxidative Stress in the Diabetic State

The occurrence of oxidative stress in diabetes has been well documented [38-40]. West reported an increase in oxidative damage in both diabetes mellitus and deficits of antioxidant defense enzymes and vitamins. It is argued that oxygen, antioxidant defenses, and cellular redox status should be regarded as central players in diabetes [41].

Chronic hyperglycemia causes increased formation of advanced glycated end products, increased glucose auto-oxidation and oxidative phosphorylation, which lead to oxidative stress. It is well established that hyperglycemia elicits an increase in ROS production, due to an increased input of reducing equivalents into the mitochondrial electron transport chain [38]. Thus, hyperglycemia-induced oxidative stress or activation of other pathways may cause tissue damage.

Mitochondrial dysfunction is considered to be a critical component in the development of diabetes mellitus such as STZ-induced diabetic rats and mice where hyperglycemia induces an acceleration of hydroxyl radical generation, and this has been correlated with the level of thiobarbituric acid (TBA) – reactive compounds as an estimation of lipoperoxidation [42, 43]. In this connection, we have demonstrated that hyperglycemia increases hydroxyl radical production in the liver of STZ-induced diabetic rats [8]. In addition, the increase in oxidative stress induced by hyperglycemia and inflammation conduces to the development of associated diseases, such as diabetic nephropathy [44, 45].

On the other hand, oxidative stress plays a pivotal role in the pathophysiology of inflammation [46] which is a critical component of the cascade of events leading to the development of diabetic complications.

### 3.2. Inflammation in the Diabetic State

Chronic hyperglycemia can directly promote an inflammatory state, where the increase in cytokines can lead to the destruction of pancreatic B cells and malfunction of the endocrine pancreas in diabetes mellitus (DM) [47].

There is evidence that autocrine insulin exerts protective anti-apoptotic effects on beta cells and inhibits the suppressor of cytokine signaling (SOCS) induced by various cytokines and leads to the apoptosis of the beta cell [48].

DM is considered an inflammatory processes [44, 49] as there is a significant increase in IL-6, IL-18, IL-1 and TNF-α in the blood of patients with this disease [50, 51]. Furthermore, chemokines (ligands 2 and 5 chemokines CCL2, CCL5 and CX3CL1), intercellular adhesion molecule-1 (ICAM-1), vascular cell adhesion molecule-1 (VCAM-1) and nuclear transcription factor kB (NFkB) are involved in the development and progression of the disease [45, 52] Our guiding hypothesis was that inflammation could be important in the development of hepatic complications in diabetes [53].

As stated above, one of the main cytokines released in diabetes inflammatory processes is TNF-α, which can activate signaling pathways associated with cell survival, apoptosis, inflammatory response and cell differentiation. The induction of the responses mediated by TNF-α occurs through the binding of the cytokine to the receptors TNF-R1 and TNF-R2. Both receptors may mediate cell death. TNF-R1 contains a death domain while TNF-R2 does not, but it would enhance the cytotoxic effects of TNF-R1. In response to inflammation and infection, TNF-α is produced primarily by immune system cells such as macrophages and lymphocytes [54, 55].

The binding of TNF-α to TNF-R1 can promote the activation of NFkB or initiate the activation of caspases, which play a major role in the execution of programmed cell death or apoptosis [56]. NFkB stimulates the expression of genes encoding cytokines (e.g. TNF-α, IL-1, IL-6, IL-2, IL-12, INF-γ and CM-CSF), cell adhesion molecules (CAMs), chemokine receptors and inducible enzymes (e.g., COX-2, iNOS). It also increases the expression of molecules involved in regulating cell proliferation, apoptosis and cell cycle progression, such as the cellular inhibitor of apoptosis protein 1 (c-IAP1), c-IAP2, TNF-receptor-associated factor 1 (TRAF-1), TRAF-2, B-cell lymphocyte/leukemia-2 (Bcl-2), Fas, c-myc and cyclin D1 [57, 58].

It has been found that high levels of glucose can cause apoptosis, in part, through activation of NFkB [59]. It has been shown that high glucose levels activate protein kinase C (PKC) pathway, NFkB and ROS [60-62]. Furthermore, cytokines and bacterial pathogens can activate iNOS and generate large concentrations of NO, through activation of NFkB [63].

This, in turn, might result in changes in glucose homeostasis which may complicate the prognosis of the disease.

## 3.3. Apoptosis in Liver in the Diabetic State

Diabetes causes an increased risk of chronic liver diseases [64] and even of acute hepatic necrosis and failure [65].

Apoptosis is a tightly regulated form of cell death in which a cell effectively partakes in its own demise. The programmed cell death is an essential physiological process required for normal development and maintenance of tissue homeostasis. Execution of the death program is characterized by morphological changes, which includes blebbing, chromatin condensation, nuclear fragmentation, loss of adhesion and rounding and cell shrinkage. Biochemical features associated with apoptosis include high molecular weight, DNA fragmentation and/or fragmentation into an oligonucleosomal ladder, phosphatidyl serine externalization, proteolytic cleavage of a number of intracellular substrates and mitochondrial permeability transition pore (MPTP) assembly [66]. Apoptotic cells are detected in organs, such as the liver, during development as well as in healthy adults. Increases in the number apoptotic cells are present in many chronic inflammatory and autoimmune diseases. The fundamental event in apoptosis is the activation of enzymes called caspases (so named because they are cysteine proteases that cleave proteins after aspartic residues). Two distinct pathways (mitochondrial and death receptor pathways) converge on caspase activation [67].

The oxidative stress and the redox state of a cell play a pivotal role in regulating apoptosis by the mitochondrial pathway [68]. The role of ROS in the induction of apoptosis is provided by several studies in which the addition of ROS in low levels induces apoptosis and the observation that various antioxidants can inhibit cell death [69-72]. Oxidative stress can lead to damage of the mitochondrial inner membrane, resulting in MPTP formation and subsequent release of cytochrome c and apoptosis inducing factor from the mitochondria. In the cytosol, cytochrome c complexes with apoptosis protease-activating factor-1 (Apaf-1) to activate procaspase 9, which in turn activates downstream effectors caspases (3, 6 and 7) [73]. Furthermore, the MPTP is regulated by the relative prevalence of anti-apoptotic (Bcl-2, Bcl-xl) or pro-apoptotic (Bad, Bax) Bcl-2 family members into the mitochondrial membrane [74].

In this connection, the results obtained from our studies demonstrate that apoptosis occurs in the diabetic liver. Importantly, we have identified that the hydroxyl radical contributes partially to mitochondrial cytochrome c release and caspase-3 activation, both of which are associated with hyperglycemia-induced liver apoptosis. The strong inhibition elicited by both Desferal (potent iron chelator) [75] and Tempol (direct scavenger of hydroxyl radicals) [76] on lipid peroxidation and apoptosis clearly establishes a connection between .OH production and both lipid peroxidation levels and apoptosis [8].

The death receptor pathway is iniciated by the binding of death receptors to their ligands, which results in the formation of an intracellular death domain (DISC: death-inducing signal complex) generated by the recruitment of two molecules: the death domain-associated TNF-R1 (TRADD: Tumor necrosis factor receptor type 1-associated death domain protein) and protein-associated death domain Fas (FADD: Fas-Associated protein with death domain). This complex also recruits procaspase-8 protein, which is activated by proteolysis. Releasing of the active fragment caspase-8 induces the activation of other caspases in the cytosol [77]. Thus, the DISC complex is responsible for the activation of the caspase cascade leading to apoptosis and/or activation of the kinase signaling pathway involved in apoptosis and JNK (c-Jun N- terminal kinase), resulting in the expression of genes through NFκB or AP-1 (activator protein-1) [78, 79]. The activation of caspase-8 that was induced by activation of the death receptor is followed by excision of Bid protein, generating an active fragment of 15 kDa, truncated Bid (Bid-t). Bid-t protein is translocated into the mitochondria and interacts with other proteins of the Bcl2 family (Bax and Bak) and induces the release of apoptogenic factors such as SMAC (second mitochondria-derived activator of caspases) / DIABLO (direct IAP protein with low pI), AIF (apoptosis inducing factor) and the release of cytochrome c into the cytosol, forming the apoptosome complex with APAF-1 and procaspase-9. In the apoptosome, procaspase-9 is proteolysed to its mature form, which then activates effector caspase-3, ultimately leading to apoptosis [80, 81].

In a research recently published by us, it is demonstrated that the diabetic state induces an increase of TNF-α and of its receptor TNF-R1 in the liver [82]. The increase of the TNF-α level in the liver of STZ-induced diabetic rats leads to a marked up-regulation of the NFkB pathway. NFkB is one of the key transcription factors involved in triggering the cascade of events that allow inflammation and different research groups have demonstrated its activation in the diabetic liver [53, 83]. The expression of inducible nitric oxide synthase (iNOS) is closely related to stimulation of NFkB. Indeed, NFkB recognition sites have been identified in the promoter region of the gene encoding for iNOS. In the liver of diabetic rats, we found an increase in TNF-α due to an increased expression of iNOS, which led to a high production of NO [82].

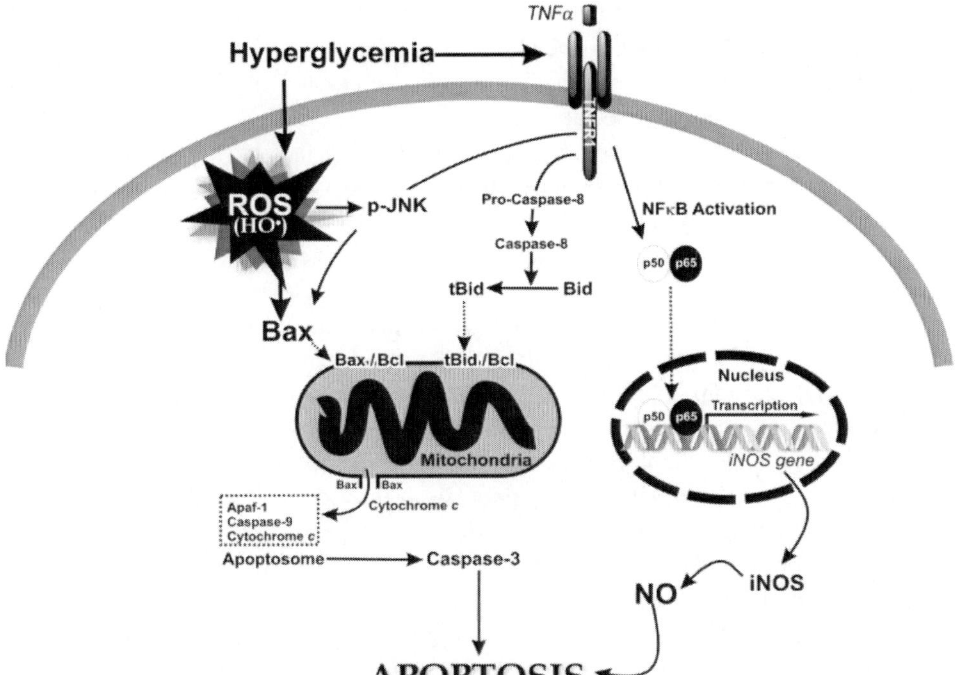


Figure 2. Proposed scheme for the mechanism involved in the hyperglycemia-induced liver apoptosis in STZ-induced insulin dependent diabetes. In the diabetic state, the increase in hepatic TNF-α induces activation of NF□B, caspase-8 and JNK, which leads to an increase in apoptotic events. Besides, hyperglycemia increases ROS levels, specifically hydroxyl radical, which initiates mitochondrial apoptosis either directly and/or by acting through BcL2 family proteins, thus inducing the formation of the mitochondrial permeability transition pore (MPTP), the release of cytochrome c and the activation of caspase 3.

Similar results have been reported in different tissues by other authors [84, 85]. We observed that the treatment with etanercept (a dimeric fusion protein that binds to TNF-α and decreases its role in disorders mediated by excess of TNF-α) [86], blocks TNF-α leading to a decrease in the expression of iNOS, which is increased in the diabetic state. Furthermore, the mentioned treatment reduces the production of NO in the liver of STZ-induced diabetic rats. It has been shown that high concentrations of glucose cause an increase in the expression of iNOS induced by cytokines [87] in rat tissues. Consistent with this, high glucose concentrations do not increase iNOS in the absence of TNF-α [82]. The inhibition of iNOS with a selective inhibitor, such as aminoguanidine, also reduced the production of TNF-α, thus evidencing an interaction between TNF-α pathway and the activity of iNOS [82]. On the other hand, in our work we described that the decrease of TNF-α level by etanercept treatment seems to completely abolish the observed activation of JNK induced by the diabetic state, thus leading to a decrease of apoptosis. Also, the administration of etanercept or AG produced a significant attenuation of both expression of activated caspase- 8 (cytosolic fraction) and Bid-t (mitochondrial fraction) when compared to STZ-induced diabetic rats.

At the light of previous knowledge and from our own results, we present a summary of the sequence of events occurring in the hepatocytes of the diabetic liver under hyperglycemic conditions (Figure 2).

## CONCLUSION

The relevance of the present review is to provide:

- First, evidences for a transient toxic effect of STZ on the hepatobiliary function. This toxic effect becomes relevant for the study, at short time, of hepatic metabolism in the experimental diabetes induced by STZ.
- Second, it provides further knowledge about the mechanisms which may contribute to the disease process in the liver during the course of an inflammatory process as is IDDM. Regulation of hepatic TNF-α levels and oxidative stress in the diabetic state could be of therapeutic relevance for the improvement or delay of the hepatic complications linked to chronic hyperglycemia.

## ACKNOWLEDGMENT

This work was supported by research grants from CONICET. We especially wish to thank Phd. Cecilia Basiglio for English revision, and also to Juan A. Monti for technical assistance.

## REFERENCES

[1] Srivastava L. M., Bora P. S., Bhatt S. D. Diabetogenic action of streptozotocin. *Trends in Pharmacological Sciences,* 1982; 3:376-378.

[2] Lenzen S. The mechanisms of alloxan- and streptozotocin-induced diabetes. *Diabetologia,* 2008; 51:216-226.

[3] Shafrir E: Diabetes in animals. In: Jr HRaDP, ed. Diabetes mellitus, theory and practice. 4th ed. Amsterdam: Elsevier, 1990; 299-340.

[4] Szkudelski T. The mechanism of alloxan and streptozotocin action in B cells of the rat pancreas. *Physiol. Res.,* 2001; 50:537-546.

[5] Ganda O. P., Rossini A. A., Like A. A. Studies on streptozotocin diabetes. *Diabetes,* 1976; 25:595-603.

[6] Katsumata K., Katsumata K., Jr., Katsumata Y. Protective effect of diltiazem hydrochloride on the occurrence of alloxan- or streptozotocin-induced diabetes in rats. *Horm. Metab. Res.,* 1992; 24:508-510.

[7] Carnovale C. E., Rodriguez Garay E. A. Reversible impairment of hepatobiliary function induced by streptozotocin in the rat. *Experientia,* 1984; 40:248-250.

[8] Frances D. E., Ronco M. T., Monti J. A., Ingaramo P. I., Pisani G. B., Parody J. P., Pellegrino J. M., et al. Hyperglycemia induces apoptosis in rat liver through the increase of hydroxyl radical: new insights into the insulin effect. *J. Endocrinol.,* 2010; 205:187-200.

[9] Portha B., Levacher C., Picon L., Rosselin G. Diabetogenic effect of streptozotocin in the rat during the perinatal period. *Diabetes,* 1974; 23:889-895.

[10] Portha B., Picon L., Rosselin G. Chemical diabetes in the adult rat as the spontaneous evolution of neonatal diabetes. *Diabetologia,* 1979; 17:371-377.

[11] Giroix M. H., Portha B., Kergoat M., Bailbe D., Picon L. Glucose insensitivity and amino-acid hypersensitivity of insulin release in rats with non-insulin-dependent diabetes. A study with the perfused pancreas. *Diabetes,* 1983; 32:445-451.

[12] Morgan N. G., Cable H. C., Newcombe N. R., Williams G. T. Treatment of cultured pancreatic B-cells with streptozotocin induces cell death by apoptosis. *Biosci. Rep.,* 1994; 14:243-250.

[13] Elsner M., Guldbakke B., Tiedge M., Munday R., Lenzen S. Relative importance of transport and alkylation for pancreatic beta-cell toxicity of streptozotocin. *Diabetologia,* 2000; 43:1528-1533.

[14] Sandler S., Swenne I. Streptozotocin, but not alloxan, induces DNA repair synthesis in mouse pancreatic islets in vitro. *Diabetologia*, 1983; 25:444-447.

[15] Heller B., Burkle A., Radons J., Fengler E., Jalowy A., Muller M., Burkart V., et al. Analysis of oxygen radical toxicity in pancreatic islets at the single cell level. *Biol. Chem. Hoppe. Seyler.*, 1994; 375:597-602.

[16] Nukatsuka M., Yoshimura Y., Nishida M., Kawada J. Importance of the concentration of ATP in rat pancreatic beta cells in the mechanism of streptozotocin-induced cytotoxicity. *J. Endocrinol.*, 1990; 127:161-165.

[17] Masiello P., Novelli M., Fierabracci V., Bergamini E. Protection by 3-aminobenzamide and nicotinamide against streptozotocin-induced beta-cell toxicity in vivo and in vitro. *Res. Commun. Chem. Pathol. Pharmacol.,* 1990; 69:17-32.

[18] Karunanayake E. H., Hearse D. J., Mellows G. Streptozotocin: its excretion and metabolism in the rat. *Diabetologia,* 1976; 12:483-488.

[19] Karunanayake E. H., Hearse D. J., Mellows G. The synthesis of [14C] streptozotocin and its distribution and excretion in the rat. *Biochem. J.,* 1974; 142:673-683.

[20] Thurston J. R., Baetz A. L., Cheville N. F., Richard J. L. Acute aflatoxicosis in guinea pigs: sequential changes in serum proteins, complement, C4, and liver enzymes and histopathologic changes. *Am. J. Vet. Res., 1980*; 41:1272-1276.

[21] Bohan A., Boyer J. L. Mechanisms of hepatic transport of drugs: implications for cholestatic drug reactions. *Semin. Liver Dis.*, 2002; 22:123-136.

[22] Russell D. W., Setchell K. D. Bile acid biosynthesis. *Biochemistry,* 1992; 31:4737-4749.

[23] Ballatori N., Truong A. T. Glutathione as a primary osmotic driving force in hepatic bile formation. *Am. J. Physiol.,* 1992; 263:G617-624.

[24] Hardison W. G., Wood C. A. Importance of bicarbonate in bile salt independent fraction of bile flow. *Am. J. Physiol.,* 1978; 235:E158-164.

[25] Alin P., Jensson H., Guthenberg C., Danielson U. H., Tahir M. K., Mannervik B. Purification of major basic glutathione transferase isoenzymes from rat liver by use of affinity chromatography and fast protein liquid chromatofocusing. *Anal. Biochem.,* 1985; 146:313-320.

[26] Cattori V., van Montfoort J. E., Stieger B., Landmann L., Meijer D. K., Winterhalter K. H., Meier P. J., et al. Localization of organic anion transporting polypeptide 4 (Oatp4) in rat liver and comparison of its substrate specificity with Oatp1, Oatp2 and Oatp3. *Pflugers Arch.,* 2001; 443:188-195.

[27] Tanaka H., Sano N., Takikawa H. Biliary excretion of phenolphthalein sulfate in rats. *Pharmacology,* 2003; 68:177-182.

[28] Erlinger S., Dhumeaux D. Mechanisms and control of secretion of bile water and electrolytes. *Gastroenterology,* 1974; 66:281-304.

[29] Carnovale C. E., Marinelli R. A., Rodriguez Garay E. A. Bile flow decrease and altered bile composition in streptozotocin-treated rats. *Biochem. Pharmacol.,* 1986; 35:2625-2628.

[30] Krenhuber H. G., Felberbauer F. X., Graf J. Is intracellular pH and/or intracellular bicarbonate a determinant of bile salt independent canalicular bile formation? The subject revisited. *Yale J. Biol. Med.,* 1997; 70:459-469.

[31] Roma M. G., Crocenzi F. A., Sanchez Pozzi E. A. Hepatocellular transport in acquired cholestasis: new insights into functional, regulatory and therapeutic aspects. *Clin. Sci. (Lond),* 2008; 114:567-588.

[32] Schein P. S., Cooney D. A., Vernon M. L. The use of nicotinamide to modify the toxicity of streptozotocin diabetes without loss of antitumor activity. *Cancer Res.,* 1967; 27:2324-2332.

[33] Carnovale C. E., Roma M. G., Monti J. A., Rodriguez Garay E. A. Studies on the mechanism of bile salt-independent bile flow impairment in streptozotocin-induced hepatotoxicity. *Toxicology,* 1991; 68:207-215.

[34] Strange R. C. Hepatic bile flow. *Physiol. Rev.,* 1984; 64:1055-1102.

[35] Carrillo M. C., Monti J. A., Grosman M. E., Rodriguez Garay E. A. Effect of pH on aflatoxin B1 transfer in the everted rat jejunum. *Toxicol. Lett.,* 1985;27:35-44.

[36] Carnovale C. E., Carrillo M. C., Grosman M. E., Monti J. A., Rodriguez Garay E. A. Intestinal transfer of sodium [14C]taurocholate in streptozotocin-treated rats. *Toxicol. Lett.,* 1988; 40:99-107.

[37] Stone J. L., Braunstein J. B., Beaty T. M., Sanders R. A., Watkins J. B., 3rd. Hepatobiliary excretion of bile acids and rose bengal in streptozotocin-induced and genetic diabetic rats. *J. Pharmacol. Exp. Ther.,* 1997; 281:412-419.

[38] Brownlee M. Biochemistry and molecular cell biology of diabetic complications. *Nature,* 2001; 414:813-820.

[39] Desco M. C., Asensi M., Marquez R., Martinez-Valls J., Vento M., Pallardo F. V., Sastre J., et al. Xanthine oxidase is involved in free radical production in type 1 diabetes: protection by allopurinol. *Diabetes,* 2002; 51:1118-1124.

[40] Matsumoto S., Koshiishi I., Inoguchi T., Nawata H., Utsumi H. Confirmation of superoxide generation via xanthine oxidase in streptozotocin-induced diabetic mice. *Free Radic. Res.,* 2003; 37:767-772.

[41] West I. C. Radicals and oxidative stress in diabetes. *Diabet Med.,* 2000; 17:171-180.

[42] Ohkuwa T., Sato Y., Naoi M. Hydroxyl radical formation in diabetic rats induced by streptozotocin. *Life Sci.,* 1995; 56:1789-1798.

[43] Winiarska K., Drozak J., Wegrzynowicz M., Fraczyk T., Bryla J. Diabetes-induced changes in glucose synthesis, intracellular glutathione status and hydroxyl free radical generation in rabbit kidney-cortex tubules. *Mol. Cell Biochem.,* 2004; 261:91-98.

[44] Alexandraki K. I., Piperi C., Ziakas P. D., Apostolopoulos N. V., Makrilakis K., Syriou V., Diamanti-Kandarakis E., et al. Cytokine secretion in long-standing diabetes mellitus type 1 and 2: associations with low-grade systemic inflammation. *J. Clin. Immunol.,* 2008; 28:314-321.

[45] Elmarakby A. A., Sullivan J. C. Relationship between oxidative stress and inflammatory cytokines in diabetic nephropathy. *Cardiovasc. Ther.,* 2012; 30:49-59.

[46] Kabe Y., Ando K., Hirao S., Yoshida M., Handa H. Redox regulation of NF-kappaB activation: distinct redox regulation between the cytoplasm and the nucleus. *Antioxid. Redox. Signal,* 2005; 7:395-403.

[47] Ahrens B. Antibodies in metabolic diseases. *N. Biotechnol.,* 2011; 28:530-537.

[48] Venieratos P. D., Drossopoulou G. I., Kapodistria K. D., Tsilibary E. C., Kitsiou P. V. High glucose induces suppression of insulin signalling and apoptosis via upregulation of endogenous IL-1beta and suppressor of cytokine signalling-1 in mouse pancreatic beta cells. *Cell Signal,* 2010; 22:791-800.

[49] Erbagci A. B., Tarakcioglu M., Coskun Y., Sivasli E., Sibel Namiduru E. Mediators of inflammation in children with type I diabetes mellitus: cytokines in type I diabetic children. *Clin. Biochem.,* 2001; 34:645-650.

[50] Esposito K., Nappo F., Marfella R., Giugliano G., Giugliano F., Ciotola M., Quagliaro L., et al. Inflammatory cytokine concentrations are acutely increased by hyperglycemia in humans: role of oxidative stress. *Circulation,* 2002; 106:2067-2072.

[51] Foss N. T., Foss-Freitas M. C., Ferreira M. A., Cardili R. N., Barbosa C. M., Foss M. C. Impaired cytokine production by peripheral blood mononuclear cells in type 1 diabetic patients. *Diabetes Metab.,* 2007; 33:439-443.

[52] Navarro-Gonzalez J. F., Muros M., Mora-Fernandez C., Herrera H., Meneses B., Garcia J. Pentoxifylline for renoprotection in diabetic nephropathy: the PREDIAN study. Rationale and basal results. *J. Diabetes Complications*, 2011; 25:314-319.

[53] Boden G., She P., Mozzoli M., Cheung P., Gumireddy K., Reddy P., Xiang X., et al. Free fatty acids produce insulin resistance and activate the proinflammatory nuclear factor-kappaB pathway in rat liver. *Diabetes,* 2005; 54:3458-3465.

[54] Littlejohn A. F., Tucker S. J., Mohamed A. A., McKay S., Helms M. J., Vandenabeele P., MacEwan D. J. Modulation by caspases of tumor necrosis factor-stimulated c-Jun N-terminal kinase activation but not nuclear factor-kappaB signaling. *Biochem. Pharmacol.,* 2003; 65:91-99.

[55] McFarlane S. M., Pashmi G., Connell M. C., Littlejohn A. F., Tucker S. J., Vandenabeele P., MacEwan D. J. Differential activation of nuclear factor-kappaB by tumour necrosis factor receptor subtypes. TNFR1 predominates whereas TNFR2 activates transcription poorly. *FEBS Lett.,* 2002; 515:119-126.

[56] Srinivasan K., Ramarao P. Animal models in type 2 diabetes research: an overview. *Indian J. Med. Res.,* 2007; 125:451-472.

[57] Joyce D., Albanese C., Steer J., Fu M., Bouzahzah B., Pestell R. G. NF-kappaB and cell-cycle regulation: the cyclin connection. *Cytokine. Growth Factor Rev.,* 2001; 12: 73-90.

[58] Yamamoto Y., Gaynor R. B. IkappaB kinases: key regulators of the NF-kappaB pathway. *Trends Biochem. Sci.*, 2004; 29:72-79.

[59] Lim J. W., Kim H., Kim K. H. NF-kappaB, inducible nitric oxide synthase and apoptosis by Helicobacter pylori infection. *Free Radic. Biol. Med.,* 2001; 31:355-366.

[60] Chen Y. W., Chenier I., Chang S. Y., Tran S., Ingelfinger J. R., Zhang S. L. High glucose promotes nascent nephron apoptosis via NF-kappaB and p53 pathways. *Am. J. Physiol. Renal Physiol.,* 2011; 300:F147-156.

[61] Karin M., Greten F. R. NF-kappaB: linking inflammation and immunity to cancer development and progression. *Nat. Rev. Immunol.,* 2005; 5:749-759.

[62] Yang W. S., Seo J. W., Han N. J., Choi J., Lee K. U., Ahn H., Lee S. K., et al. High glucose-induced NF-kappaB activation occurs via tyrosine phosphorylation of IkappaBalpha in human glomerular endothelial cells: involvement of Syk tyrosine kinase. *Am. J. Physiol. Renal Physiol.,* 2008; 294:F1065-1075.

[63] Kikutani H., Makino S. The murine autoimmune diabetes model: NOD and related strains. *Adv. Immunol.*, 1992; 51:285-322.

[64] El-Serag H. B., Tran T., Everhart J. E. Diabetes increases the risk of chronic liver disease and hepatocellular carcinoma. *Gastroenterology,* 2004; 126:460-468.

[65] El-Serag H. B., Everhart J. E. Diabetes increases the risk of acute hepatic failure. *Gastroenterology*, 2002; 122:1822-1828.

[66] Zimmermann K. C., Green D. R. How cells die: apoptosis pathways. *J. Allergy Clin. Immunol.,* 2001; 108:S99-103.

[67] Danial N. N., Korsmeyer S. J. Cell death: critical control points. *Cell,* 2004; 116: 205-219.

[68] Curtin J. F., Donovan M., Cotter T. G. Regulation and measurement of oxidative stress in apoptosis. *J. Immunol. Methods*, 2002; 265:49-72.

[69] Lennon S. V., Martin S. J., Cotter T. G. Dose-dependent induction of apoptosis in human tumour cell lines by widely diverging stimuli. *Cell Prolif.,* 1991; 24:203-214.

[70] Magowan G., Price D. J. Trophic and outgrowth-promoting effects of K(+)-induced depolarization on developing thalamic cells in organotypic culture. *Neuroscience,* 1996; 74: 1045-1057.

[71] Suzuki Y., Ono Y., Hirabayashi Y. Rapid and specific reactive oxygen species generation via NADPH oxidase activation during Fas-mediated apoptosis. *FEBS Lett.,* 1998; 425:209-212.

[72] Wolf H., Muller Y., Salmen S., Wilmanns W., Jung G. Induction of anergy in resting human T lymphocytes by immobilized anti-CD3 antibodies. *Eur. J. Immunol.,* 1994; 24: 1410-1417.

[73] Bai J., Odin J. A. Apoptosis and the liver: relation to autoimmunity and related conditions. *Autoimmun. Rev*., 2003; 2:36-42.

[74] Ronco M. T., deAlvarez M. L., Monti J., Carrillo M. C., Pisani G., Lugano M. C., Carnovale C. E. Modulation of balance between apoptosis and proliferation by lipid peroxidation (LPO) during rat liver regeneration. *Mol. Med*., 2002; 8:808-817.

[75] Knecht K. T., Mason R. P. In vivo spin trapping of xenobiotic free radical metabolites. *Arch. Biochem. Biophys*., 1993; 303:185-194.

[76] Chatterjee P. K., Cuzzocrea S., Brown P. A., Zacharowski K., Stewart K. N., Mota-Filipe H., Thiemermann C. Tempol, a membrane-permeable radical scavenger, reduces oxidant stress-mediated renal dysfunction and injury in the rat. *Kidney Int.,* 2000; 58: 658-673.

[77] Jeschke M. G., Klein D., Bolder U., Einspanier R. Insulin attenuates the systemic inflammatory response in endotoxemic rats. *Endocrinology,* 2004; 145:4084-4093.

[78] Kiechle F. L., Zhang X. Apoptosis: biochemical aspects and clinical implications. *Clin. Chim. Acta,* 2002; 326:27-45.

[79] Schattenberg J. M., Schuchmann M. Diabetes and apoptosis: liver. *Apoptosis,* 2009; 14: 1459-1471.

[80] Zhao Y., Li S., Childs E. E., Kuharsky D. K., Yin X. M. Activation of pro-death Bcl-2 family proteins and mitochondria apoptosis pathway in tumor necrosis factor-alpha-induced liver injury. *J. Biol. Chem.,* 2001; 276:27432-27440.

[81] Zimmermann K. C., Bonzon C., Green D. R. The machinery of programmed cell death. *Pharmacol. Ther.,* 2001; 92:57-70.

[82] Ingaramo P. I., Ronco M. T., Frances D. E., Monti J. A., Pisani G. B., Ceballos M. P., Galleano M., et al. Tumor necrosis factor alpha pathways develops liver apoptosis in type 1 diabetes mellitus. *Mol. Immunol.,* 2011; 48:1397-1407.

[83] Romagnoli M., Gomez-Cabrera M. C., Perrelli M. G., Biasi F., Pallardo F. V., Sastre J., Poli G., et al. Xanthine oxidase-induced oxidative stress causes activation of NF-kappaB and inflammation in the liver of type I diabetic rats. *Free Radic. Biol. Med.,* 2010; 49:171-177.

[84] Powell L. A., Warpeha K. M., Xu W., Walker B., Trimble E. R. High glucose decreases intracellular glutathione concentrations and upregulates inducible nitric oxide synthase gene expression in intestinal epithelial cells. *J. Mol. Endocrinol.,* 2004; 33:797-803.

[85] Stadler K., Bonini M. G., Dallas S., Jiang J., Radi R., Mason R. P., Kadiiska M. B. Involvement of inducible nitric oxide synthase in hydroxyl radical-mediated lipid peroxidation in streptozotocin-induced diabetes. *Free Radic. Biol. Med.,* 2008; 45:866-874.

[86] Madhusudan S., Muthuramalingam S. R., Braybrooke J. P., Wilner S., Kaur K., Han C., Hoare S., et al. Study of etanercept, a tumor necrosis factor-alpha inhibitor, in recurrent ovarian cancer. *J. Clin. Oncol.,* 2005; 23:5950-5959.

[87] Noh H., Ha H., Yu M.,R., Kang S. W., Choi K. H., Han D. S., Lee H. Y. High glucose increases inducible NO production in cultured rat mesangial cells. Possible role in fibronectin production. *Nephron,* 2002; 90:78-85.

# INDEX

## B



## C

## D

## E

## F



## G

## H



## I

## J



## K



## L



## M

## N

## Q



## R

## S



## T

## U



## V



## W



## Y

## Z



## β